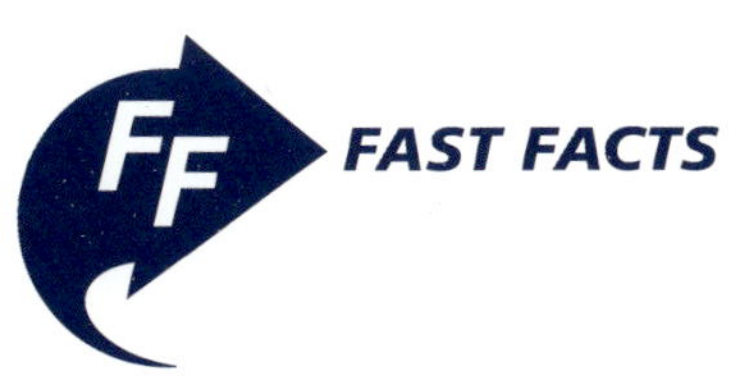


# Acute Myeloid Leukemia

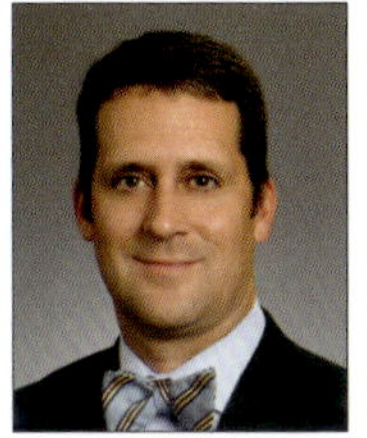

**William Blum MD**
Professor, Department of Hematology and Medical Oncology
Emory University School of Medicine
Director, Acute Leukemia Program
Winship Cancer Institute of Emory University
Atlanta, Georgia, USA

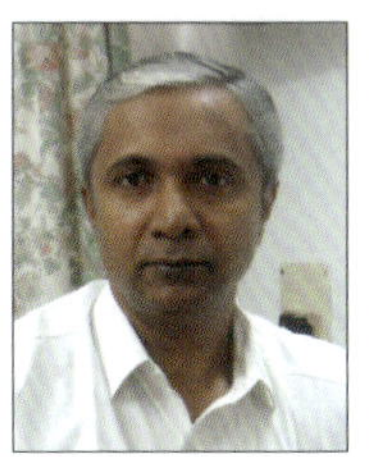

**Vikram Mathews MD DM**
Associate Director
Professor and Head
Department of Haematology
Christian Medical College
Vellore, India

**Declaration of Independence**
This book is as balanced and as practical as we can make it.
Ideas for improvement are always welcome: feedback@fastfacts.com

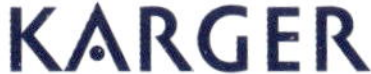

Fast Facts: Acute Myeloid Leukemia
First edition May 2018


S. Karger Publishers Limited, Elizabeth House, Queen Street,
Abingdon, Oxford OX14 3LN, UK
Tel: +44 (0)1235 523233

Book orders can be placed by telephone or via the website.
For regional distributors or to order via the website, please go to:
fastfacts.com
For telephone orders, please call +44 (0)1752 202301



A CIP record for this title is available from the British Library.

ISBN 978-1-910797-59-4

Blum W (William)
Fast Facts: Acute Myeloid Leukemia/
William Blum, Vikram Mathews

Typesetting by Thomas Bohm, User Design, Illustration and Typesetting, UK.
Printed in the UK with Xpedient Print.

Made possible by a contribution from Helsinn Healthcare S.A. Helsinn did not have any influence on the content and all items were subject to independent peer and editorial review.

## List of abbreviations

**alloHCT:** allogeneic hematopoietic cell transplantation

**AML:** acute myeloid leukemia

**APL:** acute promyelocytic leukemia

**AraC:** cytosine arabinoside (cytarabine)

**ATO:** arsenic trioxide

**ATRA:** all-*trans*-retinoic acid

**autoHCT:** autologous hematopoietic cell transplantation

**BSC:** best supportive care

**CI:** confidence interval

**CNS:** central nervous system

**CR:** complete remission

**CR1:** complete remission following induction chemotherapy

**DFS:** disease-free survival

**DIC:** disseminated intravascular coagulation

**EBMT:** European Group for Blood and Marrow Transplantation

**ELN:** European LeukemiaNet

**FAB:** French–American–British

**FDA:** US Food and Drug Administration

**G-CSF:** granulocyte colony-stimulating factor

**GO:** gemtuzumab ozogamicin

**2-HG:** 2-hydroxyglutarate

**HCT:** hematopoietic cell transplantation

**HDAC:** histone deacetylase inhibitors

**HLA:** human leukocyte antigen

**HR:** hazard ratio

**IBMTR:** International Bone Marrow Transplant Registry

**IDH:** isocitrate dehydrogenase

**ITD:** internal tandem duplications

**MDR:** multidrug resistant

**MDS:** myelodysplastic syndromes

**MFC:** multiparameter flow cytometry

**MPN:** myeloproliferative neoplasms

**MRD:** measurable residual disease

**NGS:** next-generation sequencing

**OS:** overall survival

**PBSC:** peripheral blood stem cells

**PS:** performance status

**RIC:** reduced-intensity conditioning

**RT-qPCR:** real-time quantitative polymerase chain reaction

**TCGA:** The US Cancer Genome Atlas

**TKD:** tyrosine kinase domain

**TKI:** tyrosine kinase inhibitor

**TLS:** tumor lysis syndrome

**TRM:** treatment-related mortality

**WBC:** white blood cells

**WHO:** World Health Organization

# Introduction

Acute myeloid leukemia (AML), although rare, is the most common acute leukemia in adults. Long-term survival is poor, especially in older patients (> 60 years). However, in recent years, remarkable progress has been made in our understanding of both the pathophysiology and underlying genetics of AML. As a result, at least in part, the identification of new targets for treatment is accelerating.

Four new treatments for AML have recently been approved – the first new approvals for decades; hopefully these, and other emerging therapies, will lead to a meaningful improvement in outcome for patients. New treatments such as enasidenib, which targets abnormal isocitrate dehydrogenase 2 (IDH2) in the Krebs cycle, illustrate the critical importance of understanding the cytogenetic and molecular abnormalities in individual patients, and the potential for patient benefit when these can be uniquely targeted.

This book provides a foundation for the understanding of AML, initially covering basic epidemiology, diagnosis and 'standard' treatment, then focusing on the genetics underpinning this disease, such as mutations in *IDH2*. Also highlighted is the continued need to recognize immunologic therapy (e.g. allogeneic stem cell transplantation [alloHCT]) as the best means to prevent relapse.

Chapter 1 discusses the impact of AML on populations around the world, and introduces the role of specific genetic mutations in the pathophysiology of AML. Chapter 2 describes the clinical features at presentation, and demonstrates that establishing a diagnosis is not a matter of histological appearance alone but also includes a complex process of classification based also on an individual's cytogenetic and molecular features.

Recognizing the tremendous heterogeneity of AML in a population of patients, and the unique molecular profile in an individual patient, is a crucial step in developing therapeutic strategies to improve outcomes. The new drugs recently approved, and novel approaches to treatment that are in development, offer great hope to patients. *Fast Facts: Acute Myeloid Leukemia* provides a perfect foundation for clinicians and medical students who face the challenge of keeping up to date with innovations and understanding how these are best incorporated into clinical practice.

# 1 Epidemiology, pathophysiology and etiology

Acute myeloid leukemia (AML) is a hematologic malignancy that affects the blood and bone marrow. The build up of abnormal white blood cells interferes with the production of red blood cells, platelets and white blood cells, and indirectly leads to leukemic complications of infection, fatigue and hemorrhage. Complications also arise directly from the proliferation and accumulation of immature leukemia cells, which can affect blood flow or infiltrate other organs. The pathogenesis is described in more detail on page 9.

## Epidemiology

**Incidence** data specific for AML worldwide are limited, as AML is usually included within the broader category of leukemia in epidemiology registries such as GLOBOCAN. The incidence of AML in the USA is 4.2 per 100000 per year, with an estimated 21380 new cases in 2017.[1] AML accounts for about 1.3% of all new cancer cases and 31% of all new leukemia cases.[2] In the UK in 2014, there were 3072 new cases of AML (fewer than 1% of all new cancer cases); there the incidence has risen by 28% since the early 1990s.[3] Annual incidence rates differ little between large datasets from the USA (Surveillance, Epidemiology, and End Results), the UK (Cancer Research UK), and Sweden (Swedish Acute Leukemia Registry). Data from developing countries are sparse. AML is rare compared with other cancers, but is the most common acute leukemia in adults.[1–4]

**Age, sex and ethnicity.** While AML affects all age groups, the incidence increases with advancing age (Figure 1.1), presenting at a median age of 67–69 years. AML is slightly more common in men than women, particularly in the older age groups.[4] It is more commonly diagnosed in developed countries and is more common in white than in other populations.[1–3]

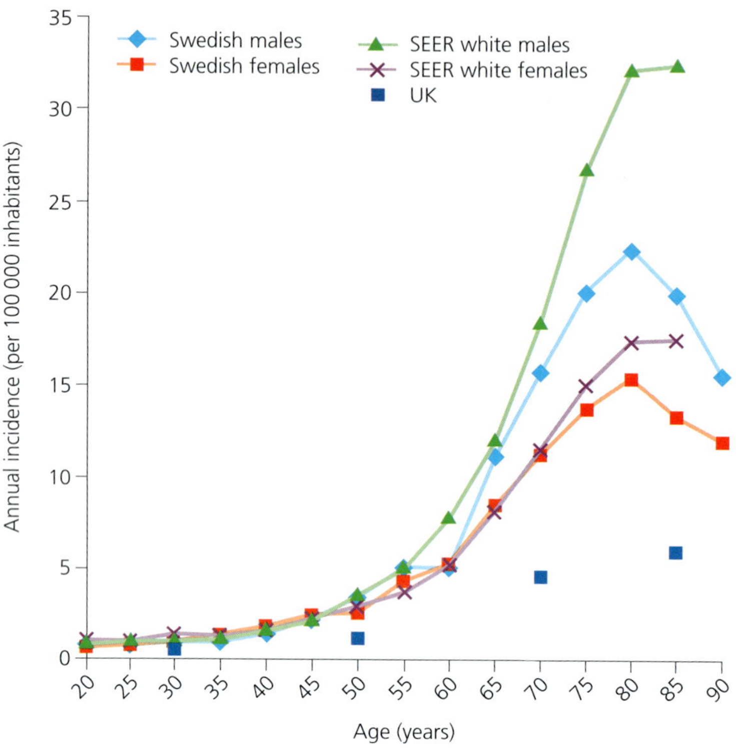


**Figure 1.1** Annual incidence of acute myeloid leukemia according to age and sex in Sweden (1997–2006), the USA (Surveillance, Epidemiology, and End Results [SEER], 2004–2008) and the UK (1987–2006; data for 20-year age intervals: 20–39, 40–59, 60–79, 80+ years). Adapted from Juliusson et al., 2012.[4]

**Survival.** AML is universally fatal if untreated. Even with treatment, patients seldom survive long term: according to US registry data, only 27% of patients survive 5 years from diagnosis. Survival is particularly poor in older patients, with fewer than 10% surviving 5 years.[5] This is attributed to a marked increase in intrinsic chemoresistance with age and a greater number of comorbidities that compromise tolerance to chemotherapy. Some older patients do not receive treatment for AML because of these concerns, although data from the Swedish Acute Leukemia Registry demonstrate that this population benefits from treatment instead of purely palliative care.[4,5] Figure 1.2 shows overall survival estimates by age group for patients in the Swedish registry.

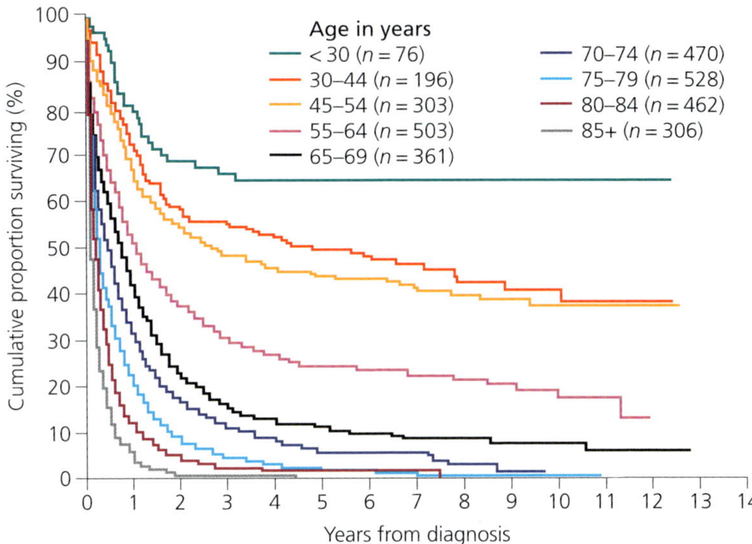


**Figure 1.2** Estimated overall survival according to age for patients diagnosed with acute myeloid leukemia in Sweden between 1997 and 2006, with follow-up in December 2008 (patients with favorable-risk acute promyelocytic leukemia were excluded). Adapted from Juliusson et al., 2012.[4]

## Pathophysiology

AML is a hematologic malignancy arising from hematopoietic progenitor (stem) cells in the bone marrow (Figure 1.3). Clonal immature myeloid progenitor cells accumulate in the blood, bone marrow and, occasionally, extramedullary tissues. While these cells can divide and proliferate, they do not differentiate (mature) into functional cells (i.e. neutrophils).

As noted above, patients experience complications directly from the accumulation of abnormal immature myeloblasts (or myeloid blasts) and indirectly from the reduction in functional myeloid cells and other mature hematopoietic elements. The leukemic involvement of the bone marrow often results in pancytopenia – patients may present with cytopenias in all hematopoietic cell lineages. Patients typically require transfusions of red blood cells and platelets and are at risk of life-threatening infectious complications due to neutropenia. Most patients with AML die from infection or, to a lesser extent, hemorrhage.

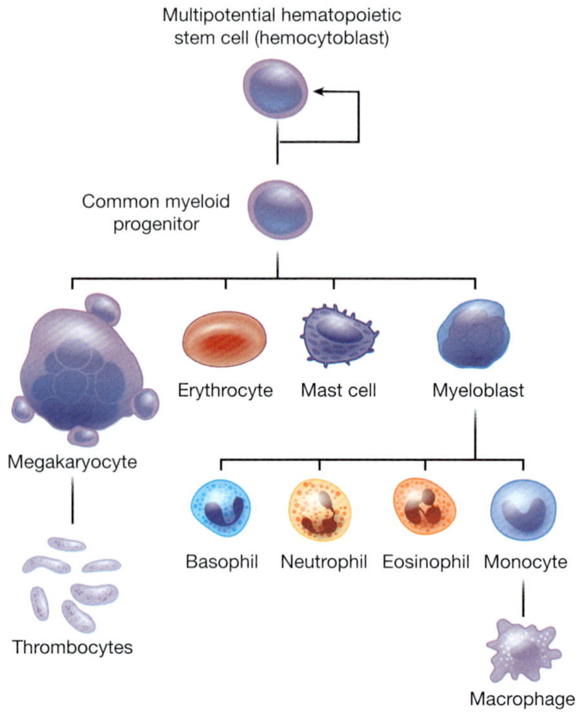


**Figure 1.3** The process of hematopoiesis (formation of blood cells). Acute myeloid leukemia affects the myeloid rather than the lymphoid lineage (not shown), and can develop from myeloid stem cells (i.e. the common myeloid progenitor) or myeloblasts. The proliferation of immature myeloblasts in the bone marrow reduces the formation of normal white blood cells, erythrocytes (red blood cells) and thrombocytes (platelets), ultimately resulting in pancytopenia.

## The role of genetics

Advances in genetics have dramatically improved our understanding of the pathophysiology of AML. Although in-depth understanding of the relationship between a specific genetic mutation and a specific pathophysiological or clinical feature is clear in only a few cases, this is slowly changing. One such example is the association of the *PML–RARA* fusion gene with acute promyelocytic leukemia (APL), which is a subtype of AML (see Tables 2.2 and 2.3). The *PML–RARA* fusion gene is typically detected as a chromosomal rearrangement: t(15;17)(q22;q21).

Patients with APL have a high risk for fatal hemorrhage due to disseminated intravascular coagulation (DIC), the consequence of a halt in myeloid differentiation that is mediated by the *PML–RARA* fusion gene. The *PML–RARA* fusion gene encodes a chimeric protein that disrupts various cellular processes, including nuclear body formation and apoptosis, adversely affecting normal myeloid development. In normal cells, *RARA* encodes a member of the nuclear hormone receptor family of transcription factors; *PML* is important in controlling proliferation and apoptosis, among other processes. The PML–RARA fusion protein suppresses gene transcription and blocks differentiation beyond the promyelocyte stage, resulting in the accumulation of malignant promyelocytes seen in APL. Degranulation of promyelocytes contributes to the development of DIC in patients with APL, putting them at risk for hemorrhage. The complex role of the PML–RARA fusion protein in modulating cellular functions is largely, and remarkably, understood.[6] Treatment of APL is unique and ultimately capitalizes on these unique pathophysiological findings (though clinical advances preceded genetic understanding in this case; see pages 49–50 for the treatment of APL).

Our understanding of the relationships between other genetic lesions and the pathophysiology of AML is limited but growing rapidly; it is hoped that understanding these relationships will identify new drug targets and enable novel therapies to be developed (e.g. midostaurin and enasidenib, see Chapter 3).

**Genetic sequencing studies** suggest that most cases of AML arise from a limited number of mutations that accumulate with age. For example, The Cancer Genome Atlas (TCGA) (cancergenome.nih.gov) and other databases have shown that up to 5–6% of healthy individuals over 70 years of age have blood cells that contain potentially 'premalignant' mutations that are associated with clonal expansion (reviewed in TCGA Research Network 2013[7]). However, the final insults that subsequently direct premalignant blood cells to become leukemic are many and remain poorly understood.

Sequencing data demonstrate the surprising finding that AML is associated with far fewer mutations than most other adult cancers: adults with AML have an average of 13 genetic mutations,[7] in stark contrast to melanoma and non-small-cell lung cancer, which typically have several hundred, as illustrated in Figure 1.4.[8]

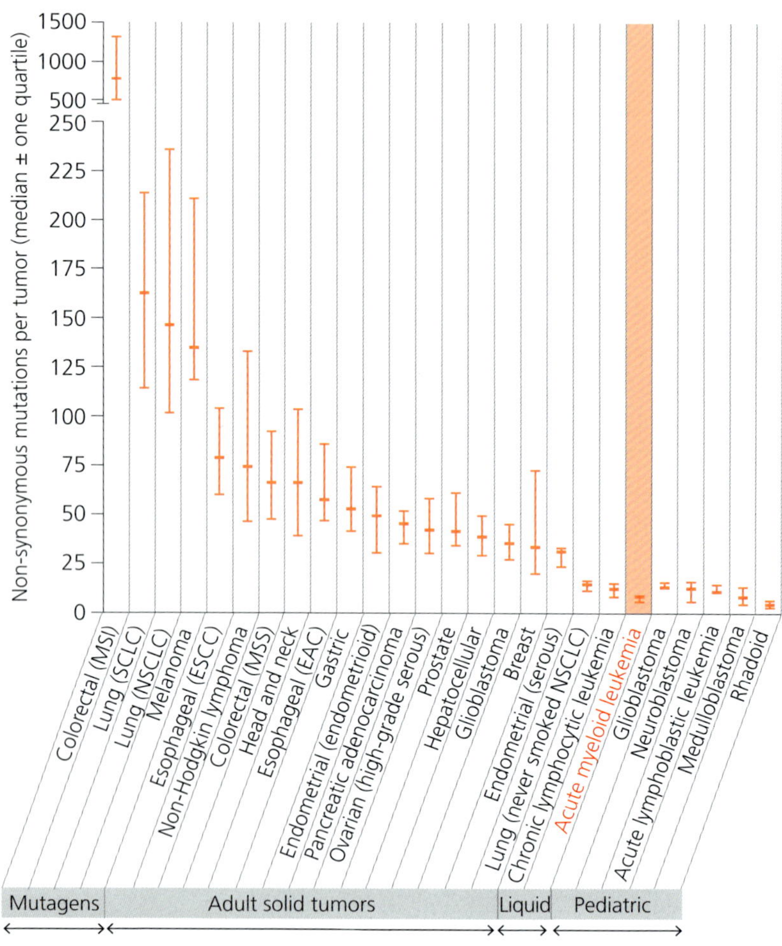


**Figure 1.4** Median numbers of non-synonymous (missense or nonsense) mutations per tumor in a variety of tumor types. The top and bottom of each bar indicate the 25% and 75% quartiles. EAC, esophageal adenocarcinoma; ESCC, esophageal squamous cell carcinoma; MSI, microsatellite instability; MSS, microsatellite stable; NSCLC, non-small-cell lung cancer; SCLC, small-cell lung cancer. Adapted from Vogelstein et al., 2013.[9]

TCGA has also shown that, on average, only five of 13 mutations found in a typical patient with AML are in genes known to be frequently mutated in AML. Despite the relatively low number of known mutations, there is tremendous heterogeneity in the types of mutation found in patients with AML. Furthermore, genetic analysis of serial samples from patients suggests that the pathogenesis of the disease is (at least in most cases) not rooted in a single mutation but in complex relationships between the accumulated (but limited number of) mutations.[7,8,10,11]

Several datasets have grouped mutations into categories in an attempt to understand these relationships. For example, TCGA reported that almost all samples had at least one mutation in one of nine categories defined according to biological function and that are thought to have a role in the pathogenesis of AML (Table 1.1).

Figure 1.5 shows the frequency of mutation for the most commonly mutated genes, which include *FLT3*, *NPM1*, *DNMT3A*, *IDH2* and *IDH1*, in a group of 200 patients with newly diagnosed AML.

The circos plot in Figure 1.6 shows the complex relationship between mutations in patients with AML. Some mutated genes are frequently (and typically) observed in the presence of other specific gene mutations, such as *NPM1* with *FLT3* (red ribbon); other gene mutations are mutually exclusive, such as *IDH1*, *IDH2* and *TET2*.

TABLE 1.1

**Frequency of genetic mutations in acute myeloid leukemia**

| Location of mutation | % of cases |
|---|---|
| Activated signaling genes | 59 |
| Genes related to DNA methylation | 44 |
| Chromatin-modifying genes | 30 |
| Nucleophosmin gene (*NPM1*) | 27 |
| Myeloid-transcription factor genes | 22 |
| Transcription factor fusions | 18 |
| Tumor suppressor genes | 16 |
| Spliceosome complex genes | 14 |
| Cohesin-complex genes | 13 |

Data from The Cancer Genome Atlas Research Network, 2013.[7]

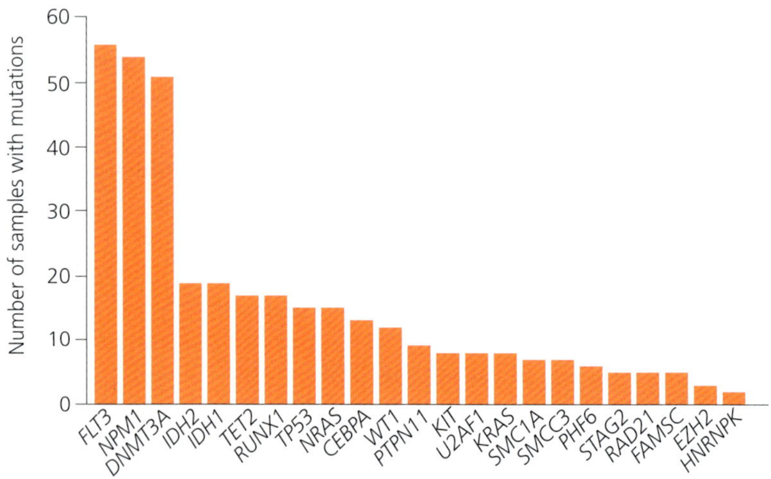


**Figure 1.5** Significant mutations in acute myeloid leukemia (AML), based on analysis of the genomes from 200 adults with AML, using whole-genome sequencing (50 genomes) or whole-exome sequencing (150), together with RNA and microRNA sequencing and DNA methylation analysis. Adapted from The Cancer Genome Atlas Research Network, 2013.[7]

**Even in a single patient, all AML cells are not equal.** Genetic sequencing studies have shown that relevant genetic variation occurs within the bone marrow cells from an individual patient with AML. Each group of cells with a shared mutation profile is called a clone; typically patients have one dominant clone and several smaller subclones. The presence of genetically different clones and subclones of myeloid blasts helps explain why a single patient may achieve remission but then experience relapse with more-resistant disease – sensitive clones are eliminated by chemotherapy, whereas surviving clones are more resistant to further rounds of chemotherapy; this is illustrated conceptually in Figure 1.7.[11] One clone may be eliminated over time (and following treatment), whereas another may persist or emerge with additional novel mutations. Figure 1.8 illustrates clonal evolution in an actual patient. Mutational analyses like these explain why patients with morphologically similar leukemias may experience vastly different clinical outcomes.[11]

Sequencing studies suggest that the development of individualized therapies that target unique mutations in selected patients, rather than a 'one way fits all' chemotherapy approach (described in

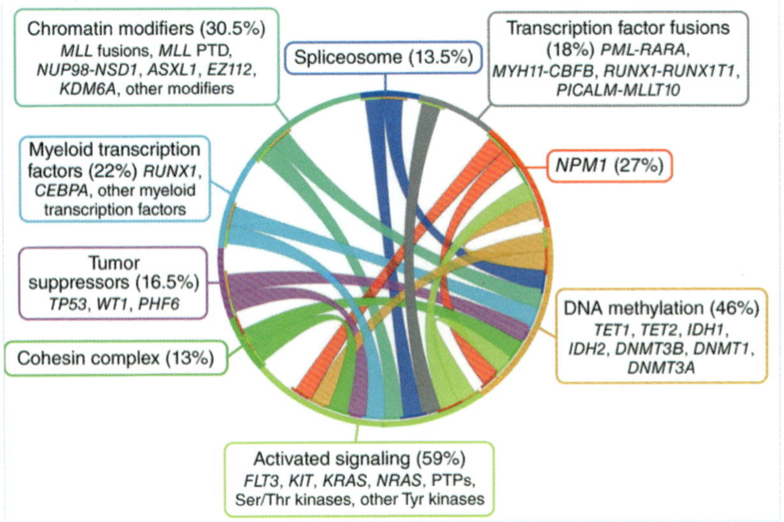


**Figure 1.6** A circos plot for acute myeloid leukemia (AML), showing the complex patterns of cooperation and mutual exclusivity between the nine functional categories identified for mutated genes. Ribbons connecting distinct categories of gene abnormalities reflect the associations between mutations in different pathways; mutually exclusive alterations may exist in areas that are not connected. Each patient with AML may have several gene mutations in different functional categories. PTD, partial tandem duplication; PTPs, protein tyrosine phosphatases. Reproduced with permission from Chen et al., 2013.[12]

Chapter 3), may improve outcomes for patients with AML. Several recent successful examples of this treatment approach are discussed in detail in Chapter 3. However, it is increasingly recognized that, in most patients, several subclones (oligoclonal) rather than a single clone contribute to the leukemia. This genetic diversity, even in a single patient, may limit the effectiveness of monotherapy with targeted agents and calls for a multitargeted approaches, including combinations with conventional chemotherapy. The use of targeted therapies to improve disease control before the use of potentially curative immunologic and decidedly non-targeted therapy (e.g. allogeneic hematopoietic cell transplantation, see Chapter 3) is another area of ongoing research.

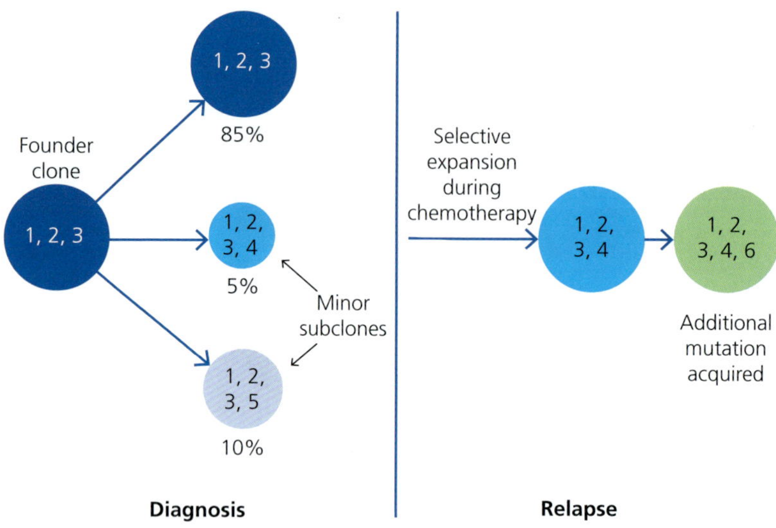


**Figure 1.7** Clonal heterogeneity in acute myeloid leukemia (AML). In this example, three AML clones were identified at diagnosis. The founder clone contains mutations 1, 2 and 3 and is the major clone (representing 85% of the total leukemic cell population). Two additional minor subclones were identified that contain at least one additional mutation (mutations 4 and 5). During chemotherapy, there is selective expansion of one of the minor subclones and acquisition of further mutations (represented as mutation 6), detected at the time of relapse. Adapted from Link, 2012.[13]

## Etiology

Most cases of AML are idiopathic, arising in previously healthy individuals with no (or unknown) genetic predisposition. Advancing age is the main risk factor for AML, as noted above and described by TCGA, but a number of other risk factors contribute to the development of AML in some patients. These include familial risk, environmental exposure to chemicals, drugs or ionizing radiation, and antecedent hematologic disorders such as myelodysplastic syndromes (MDS) or myeloproliferative neoplasms (MPN).

**Familial risk.** Although most cases of AML are not familial, it is now clear that myeloid neoplasms with germline predisposition (e.g. an inherited risk) are more frequent than has been recognized previously.

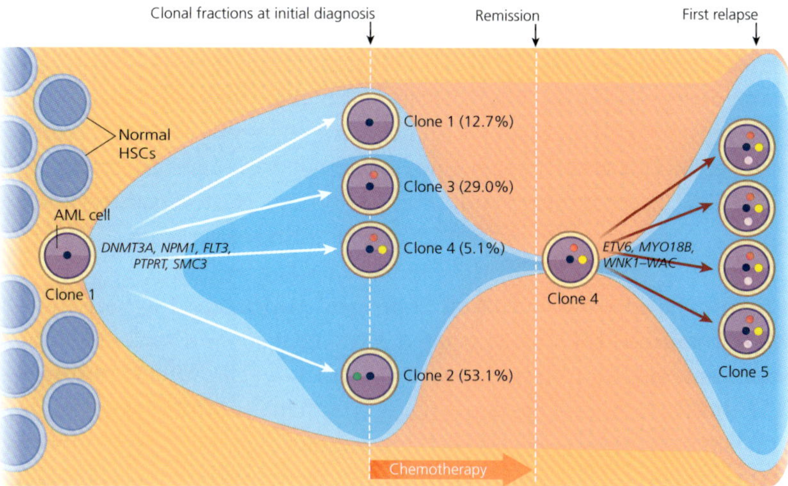


**Figure 1.8** An example of clonal evolution. In this case, the founding clone (which contains mutations of ***DNMT3A***, ***NPM1***, ***PTPRT***, ***SMC3*** and ***FLT3***). At relapse, a subclone acquires additional mutations (***ETV6***, ***MYO18B*** and ***WNK1-WAC*** fusion) and becomes the dominant clone. HSC, hematopoietic stem cells. Adapted from Ding et al., 2012.[14]

Myeloid neoplasms with germline predisposition – that is, AML and related disorders that arise in the setting of an inherited genetic mutation which puts the patient at increased risk for developing the disease – are an important component of the forthcoming revision to the World Health Organization classification of AML (see Table 2.3). Germline mutations associated with an increased risk of developing a myeloid neoplasm occur in the *CEBPA*, *DDX41*, *RUNX1*, *ANKRD26*, *ETV6* and *GATA2* genes, among others.[15]

Myeloid neoplasms with germline predisposition are a feature of several well-described clinical syndromes, including disorders of bone marrow failure (e.g. Fanconi anemia, Shwachman–Diamond syndrome, Diamond–Blackfan anemia) and telomere biology (e.g. dyskeratosis congenita). Likewise, several genetic syndromes with aberrations of somatic cell chromosome complement, such as Down syndrome with trisomy 21, are associated with an increased incidence of AML. Down syndrome-associated AML in young children (< 4 years) is typically of the acute megakaryocytic subtype (see Table 2.2 for the different morphologic subtypes) and is associated with a mutation in the *GATA1* gene. Affected patients have favorable clinical outcomes but require lower doses of chemotherapy because of higher treatment-related toxicities. Inherited diseases with defective DNA repair (e.g. Fanconi anemia, Bloom syndrome and ataxia telangiectasia) are also associated with AML. Each of these syndromes has unique clinical features and atypical toxicities after chemotherapy, requiring expert care.

**Chemical and environmental exposure.** Anticancer drugs are the leading cause of therapy-associated AML. Leukemias associated with topoisomerase II inhibitors typically occur 1–3 years after exposure; AML blasts in affected patients have a particular morphologic appearance with monocytic features. Patients who develop monocytic AML after exposure to topoisomerase II inhibitors often also have a particular chromosomal abnormality that involves the long arm of chromosome 11 (11q23 rearrangements occur in AML and may be seen with many other partner chromosomes).

Alkylating agents may also cause leukemias, on average 4–6 years after exposure; affected individuals often have abnormalities in many cells lines (multilineage dysplasia) and monosomy/aberrations in chromosomes 5 and 7.

Exposure to ionizing radiation, benzene, chloramphenicol, phenylbutazone and other drugs, although rare, may result in bone marrow failure that evolves into AML.

**Myelodysplastic syndromes/myeloproliferative neoplasms.** Several disorders of myeloid cells are related to AML and are broadly classified as MDS and MPN, with tremendous heterogeneity within each group. Detailed description of these disorders is beyond the scope of this book, but it is important to understand that MDS or MPN may progress to AML, a condition which is referred to as secondary AML or AML arising from an antecedent hematologic disorder. The risk of progression of MDS to AML can be estimated based on the proportion of blasts in the marrow (MDS is defined as < 20% blasts), cytopenias, karyotype and other factors. MPN are further subclassified into familiar terms of polycythemia vera, essential thrombocythemia and chronic myelogenous leukemia, as well as other disorders such as mastocytosis and eosinophilic disorders associated with abnormalities of *PDGFA/B* or *FGFR1*, among others.

**Key points – epidemiology, pathophysiology and etiology**

- Acute myeloid leukemia (AML) is a relatively rare cancer. It is due to proliferation of immature myeloid cells, which interfere with the production of normal red blood cells, white blood cells and platelets. Patients typically require transfusion support and are at risk for potentially fatal infection. AML is uniformly fatal without treatment.
- AML is the most common acute leukemia in older adults, with median age at diagnosis of 67–69 years.
- Long-term survival of patients with AML is poor: about a quarter of patients survive 5 years but only 10% of older patients.
- Our understanding of the genetic basis for AML is improving. A small number of mutations are seen in the typical AML patient; the mutation profile of an individual patient may change over time.
- Most cases of AML are idiopathic; however, prior exposure to topoisomerase II inhibitors and alkylating agents increases the risk of AML.
- Inherited risk is uncommon but is likely to be more frequent than is currently understood.

## References


1. NIH NCI. Cancer Stat Facts: Acute Myeloid Leukemia (AML). https://seer.cancer.gov/statfacts/html/amyl.html. Last accessed 21 August 2017.

2. American Cancer Society. Cancer Facts & Figures, 2017. https://www.cancer.org/content/dam/cancer-org/research/cancer-facts-and-statistics/annual-cancer-facts-and-figures/2017/cancer-facts-and-figures-2017.pdf.

3. Cancer Research UK. Acute myeloid leukaemia statistics. www.cancerresearchuk.org/health-professional/cancer-statistics/statistics-by-cancer-type/leukaemia-aml. Last accessed 21 August 2017.

4. Juliusson G, Lazarevic V, Horstedt AS et al. Acute myeloid leukemia in the real world: why population-based registries are needed. *Blood* 2012;119:3890–9.

5. Oran B, Weisdorf DJ. Survival for older patients with acute myeloid leukemia: a population-based study. *Haematologica* 2012;97:1916–24.

6. Ablain J, Rice K, Soilihi H et al. Activation of a promyelocytic leukemia-tumor protein 53 axis underlies acute promyelocytic leukemia cure. *Nat Med* 2014;20:167–74.

7. TCGA Research Network, Ley TJ, Miller C et al. Genomic and epigenomic landscapes of adult de novo acute myeloid leukemia. *N Engl J Med* 2013;368:2059–74.

8. Alexandrov LB, Nik-Zainal S, Wedge DC et al. Signatures of mutational processes in human cancer. *Nature* 2013;500:415–21.

9. Vogelstein B, Papadopoulos N, Velculescu V et al. Cancer genome landscapes. *Science* 2013;339:1546–58.

10. Papaemmanuil E, Gerstung M, Bullinger L et al. Genomic classification and prognosis in acute myeloid leukemia. *N Engl J Med* 2016;374:2209–21.

11. Welch JS, Ley TJ, Link DC et al. The origin and evolution of mutations in acute myeloid leukemia. *Cell* 2012;150:264–78.

12. Chen S-J, Shen Y, Chen Z. A panoramic view of acute myeloid leukemia. *Nat Genet* 2013;45:486–587.

13. Link D. Molecular genetics of AML. *Best Pract Res Clin Haematol* 2012;25:409–12.

14. Ding L, Ley TJ, Larson DE et al. Clonal evolution in relapsed acute myeloid leukaemia revealed by whole-genome sequencing. *Nature* 2012;481:506–10.

15. Brown AL, Churpek JE, Malcovati L et al. Recognition of familial myeloid neoplasia in adults. *Semin Hematol* 2017;54:60–8.

# 2 Diagnosis

## Clinical presentation

**Symptoms.** Patients with acute myeloid leukemia (AML) usually present with vague symptoms that are consequences of pancytopenia. Typically, the onset of symptoms is no more than 3 months before diagnosis. Fatigue is a common first symptom (Table 2.1), often accompanied by anorexia and weight loss. Fever or infection is the initial symptom in approximately 10% of patients, and 5% have signs of abnormal hemostasis (beyond minor bleeding and easy bruising). Bone pain, lymphadenopathy, non-specific cough, headache and diaphoresis (excessive sweating) may also occur. Bone pain, typically vaguely localized to the pelvis or back, is also a frequent symptom.

Rarely, patients present with symptoms due to extramedullary leukemia (i.e. outside the blood and marrow), such as myeloid sarcoma (a tumor mass consisting of myeloid blasts); AML may infiltrate skin, lymph nodes, the gastrointestinal tract, soft tissue or testes. Patients who present with isolated myeloid sarcoma typically develop blood and/or marrow involvement quickly thereafter. Central nervous system (CNS) involvement is uncommon in AML (approximately 5% of cases, in contrast to acute lymphoblastic leukemia where CNS involvement is common).

**Physical findings.** Fever, infection and hemorrhage are often present at the time of diagnosis. Splenomegaly, hepatomegaly and lymphadenopathy may also be present but are relatively uncommon. Hemorrhagic complications are most commonly and classically found in acute promyelocytic leukemia (APL). Affected patients often present with disseminated intravascular coagulation (DIC)-associated hemorrhage and may have intracranial hemorrhage or bleeding at other sites. Thrombosis is a less frequent but well-recognized feature of APL. Bleeding associated with coagulopathy may also occur in monocytic AML, or with extreme degrees of leukocytosis or thrombocytopenia in other morphologic subtypes.

TABLE 2.1

**Initial diagnostic evaluation and management of adults with AML**

| | |
|---|---|
| History | Fatigue or poor exercise tolerance (anemia)<br>Minor or major hemorrhage (DIC, thrombocytopenia)<br>Fevers or recurrent infections (neutropenia)<br>Headache, vision changes, non-focal neurologic abnormalities (CNS leukemia or bleed)<br>Early satiety (splenomegaly)<br>Family history of AML (germline predisposition; Fanconi, Bloom, Kostmann syndromes; ataxia telangiectasia)<br>History of cancer (exposure to alkylating agents, radiation or topoisomerase II inhibitors)<br>Occupational exposure (radiation, benzene, petroleum products, paint, smoking, pesticides) |
| Physical examination | Performance status (prognostic factor)<br>Ecchymosis and oozing from IV sites (DIC, possible acute promyelocytic leukemia)<br>Fever and tachycardia (signs of infection)<br>Papilledema, retinal infiltrates, cranial nerve abnormalities (CNS leukemia)<br>Poor dentition, dental abscesses<br>Gingival hypertrophy (leukemic infiltration, most common in monocytic leukemia)<br>Skin infiltration or nodules (leukemia infiltration, most common in monocytic leukemia)<br>Lymphadenopathy, splenomegaly, hepatomegaly (relatively uncommon in AML)<br>Back pain, lower extremity weakness (spinal granulocytic sarcoma, most likely in patients with the t(8;21) chromosome abnormality) |

CONTINUED

TABLE 2.1 (CONTINUED)

**Initial diagnostic evaluation and management of adults with AML**

| | |
|---|---|
| Laboratory and radiology studies | Complete blood count with manual differential cell count |
| | Chemistry tests (electrolytes, creatinine, BUN, calcium, phosphorus, uric acid, hepatic enzymes, bilirubin, LDH, amylase, lipase) |
| | Clotting studies (prothrombin time, partial thromboplastin time, fibrinogen, D-dimer) |
| | Viral serologies (CMV, HSV-1, varicella zoster virus) |
| | Red blood cell count, type and screen |
| | HLA typing for potential allogeneic HCT |
| | Bone marrow aspirate and biopsy (morphology, cytogenetics, flow cytometry, molecular studies, tissue banking–cryopreservation of viable leukemia cells) |
| | Myocardial function (echocardiogram or MUGA scan) |
| | Posteroanterior and lateral chest radiograph |
| | Placement of central venous access device |
| Interventions for specific patients | Dental evaluation (for those with poor dentition) |
| | Lumbar puncture (for those with symptoms of CNS involvement) |
| | Screening brain/spine MRI (for patients with headache, cranial nerve palsies, back pain, lower extremity weakness, paresthesias) |
| | Social work referral for patient and family psychosocial support |
| Counseling for all patients | Provide patients with information regarding their disease and genetics, financial counseling, support group contacts |

AML, acute myeloid leukemia; BUN, blood urea nitrogen; CMV, cytomegalovirus; CNS, central nervous system; DIC, disseminated intravascular coagulation; HLA, human leukocyte antigen; HCT, hematopoietic cell transplantation; HSV, herpes simplex virus; IV, intravenous; LDH, lactate dehydrogenase; MRI, magnetic resonance imaging; MUGA, multigated acquisition.

Modified from Kasper et al. *Harrison's Principles of Internal Medicine* (2015).[1]

Retinal hemorrhage due to thrombocytopenia and extreme leukocytosis is detected in approximately 15% of patients. Infiltration of the gingiva, skin, soft tissues or meninges (CNS) with leukemic blasts at diagnosis is infrequent but characteristic of the monocytic subtypes (see Tables 2.2 and 2.3) and those with 11q23 chromosomal abnormalities.

### Hematologic findings

***Red blood cells.*** Anemia is usually present at diagnosis but is not severe and is usually normocytic and normochromic (the size of red blood cells and level of hemoglobin are within normal limits). Decreased erythropoiesis often results in a reduced reticulocyte (immature red blood cell) count, and red blood cell survival may be shortened through accelerated destruction. Hemorrhage may rarely contribute to the anemia.

***White blood cells (WBC).*** The median presenting WBC count is about 15 000/μL (compared with a normal range of 4500–10 000/μL) but lower counts are commonly seen in older patients and in those with an antecedent hematologic disorder such as myelodysplastic syndromes or myeloproliferative neoplasms (see pages 18–19).

The predominant WBC is the myeloid blast. Occasionally, patients may present with no detectable leukemic cells in the blood. Extreme leukocytosis (> 100 000/μL, 'hyperleukocytosis') occurs in about 20% of cases.

On peripheral blood smears, the cytoplasm of the myeloid blast often contains primary (non-specific) granules, and the nucleus shows fine, lacy chromatin, with one or more nucleoli characteristic of immature cells. The presence of abnormal rod-shaped granules called Auer rods (Figure 2.1) on light microscopy of a blood smear or bone aspirate indicates a diagnosis of AML. Additionally, the morphology in some AML subsets is distinctly different and strongly suggests diagnosis of a particular subtype; however, this will need to be confirmed by a combination of additional diagnostic tests, such as cytochemistry, immunophenotyping, karyotype and molecular methods. For example, the myeloblasts in APL are classically hypergranular with clusters of Auer rods (called faggot cells) with a bi-lobed or reniform nucleus. While these features strongly suggest a diagnosis of APL, the final diagnosis will require demonstration of the

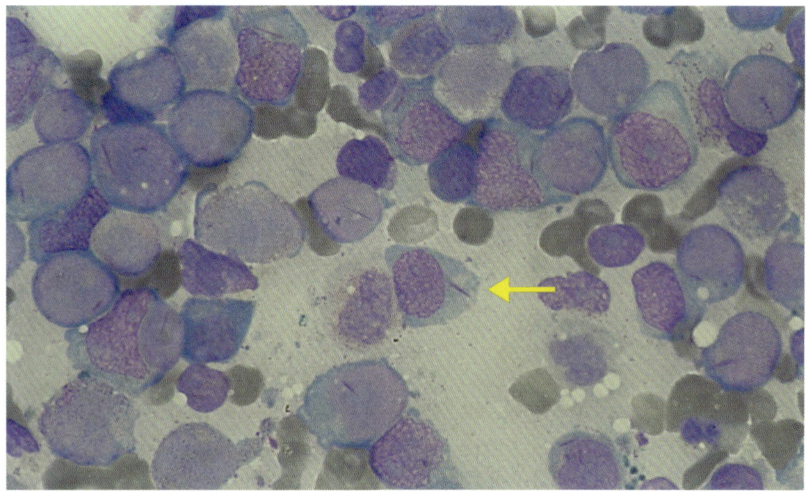

**Figure 2.1** Bone marrow aspirate from a patient with acute myeloid leukemia (AML), showing several myoblasts containing Auer rods, which are diagnostic of AML. May–Grünwald–Giemsa stain. Source: Paulo Henrique Orlandi Mourao. Creative Commons Attribution-ShareAlike 3.0 Unported (CC BY-SA 3.0) (https://creativecommons.org/licenses/by-sa/3.0/deed.en).

appropriate molecular abnormality by either karyotyping or other molecular methods.

***Platelets.*** Most patients present with at least mild thrombocytopenia (below the normal lower limit of 150 000/μL); about 25% have severe thrombocytopenia, with platelet counts below 25 000/μL.

## Differential diagnosis

Many bone marrow disorders present with pancytopenia and its attendant signs and symptoms. Highest in the differential diagnosis of pancytopenia due to acute leukemia (myeloid or lymphoblastic) are other hematologic cancers with marrow infiltration, and bone marrow failure syndromes such as aplastic anemia. Myeloproliferative disorders with bone marrow fibrosis can also present similarly. Rarely, pancytopenia caused by the displacement of hemopoietic bone marrow tissue by fibrosis, tumor or granuloma (called myelophthisis) may mimic acute leukemia. Examples include solid organ cancers with extensive marrow involvement, and granulomatous disease such as tuberculosis. However, acute leukemia is the appropriate diagnosis in patients with circulating blasts visualized on light microscopy. The circulating myeloid blasts contain Auer rods. Auer rods are not seen in lymphoblastic leukemia; their presence confirms a diagnosis of myeloid leukemia.

## Pretreatment evaluation

Once a diagnosis of AML is suspected, cytogenetic and genetic tests are required to aid rapid diagnosis, assess prognosis and to inform the best approach to treatment. Initial assessments should evaluate the functional integrity of the cardiovascular, pulmonary, hepatic and renal systems, and patients should also be evaluated for infection and DIC. Preparation for transfusion of blood or platelets requires blood type and crossmatch to be determined, and human leukocyte antigen (HLA) testing is required early in the treatment course (before chemotherapy) in consideration of future allogeneic hematopoietic cell transplantation.

**Cytogenetics** has been a part of AML diagnosis for several decades, and typically requires bone marrow for successful testing (the increased number of proliferating cells in marrow yields better results than blood for karyotype analysis).

**Genetic testing** (from blood or marrow) continues to evolve in both complexity and number of tests, and should include at least *FLT3* (with allelic ratio), *NPM1*, *CEBPA* (bi-allelic), *IDH1*, *IDH2* and *TP53*. Note that the European LeukemiaNet (ELN) recommendations do not include *IDH1* and *IDH2* (although this might be expected to change given the advent of treatments targeted at the encoded proteins); the World Health Organization (WHO) classification also recognizes *RUNX1*- and *ASXL1*-mutated AML as distinct entities.

**Histology.** The diagnosis of AML is based on a finding of 20% or more myeloid blasts by histology, cytochemistry or (more commonly) flow cytometry. However, this criterion is not required for diagnosis if any of the following recurrent cytogenetic abnormalities is present: t(15;17), t(8;21), inv(16) or t(16;16).

TABLE 2.2

**The FAB classification of acute myeloid leukemia[2]**

| Subtype | Name |
|---|---|
| M0 | Undifferentiated acute myeloblastic leukemia |
| M1 | Acute myeloblastic leukemia with minimal maturation |
| M2 | Acute myeloblastic leukemia with maturation |
| M3 | Acute promyelocytic leukemia |
| M4 | Acute myelomonocytic leukemia |
| M4eos | Acute myelomonocytic leukemia with eosinophilia |
| M5 | Acute monocytic leukemia |
| M6 | Acute erythroid leukemia |
| M7 | Acute megakaryocytic leukemia |

Note that this system has been superseded by the World Health Organization and European LeukemiaNet classifications described in Tables 2.3 and 2.4, respectively, but is still useful for understanding the disease.
FAB, French–American–British

## Classification

Historically, the diagnosis and classification of AML was based on the French–American–British (FAB) criteria, which assigned patients to one of eight groups, designated M0–M7, based on morphologic and cytochemical features (Table 2.2). Essentially, M0–M5 describe stages of myeloid maturation; M6 and M7 describe erythroid leukemia and megakaryocytic leukemia, respectively. The FAB classification has been superseded by the WHO classification (Table 2.3) and the ELN risk stratification (Table 2.4), which include highly relevant cytogenetic and genetic aberrations. However, morphologic description using the FAB terminology is still a common feature of clinical discussion among clinicians and with patients.

**Cytogenetic analysis** of leukemic cells provides important independent prognostic information and is a feature of both the WHO and ELN systems. The prognostic categories using cytogenetics are 'favorable', 'intermediate' and 'adverse' risk, based on the presence of

TABLE 2.3

**The World Health Organization 2016 classification of acute myeloid leukemia (AML) and related neoplasms***

**AML with recurrent genetic abnormalities**

AML with t(8;21)(q22;q22); *RUNX1–RUNX1T1*

AML with inv(16)(p13.1q22) or t(16;16)(p13.1;q22); *CBFB–MYH11*

Acute promyelocytic leukemia with *PML–RARA* (see page 10–11)

AML with t(9;11)(p21.3;q23.3); *MLLT3–KMT2A*

AML with t(6;9)(p23;q34.1); *DEK-NUP214*

AML with inv(3)(q21.3q26.2) or t(3;3)(q21.3;q26.2); *GATA2, MECOM*

AML (megakaryoblastic) with t(1;22)(p13.3;q13.3); *RBM15-MKL1*

AML with mutated *NPM1*

AML with bi-allelic mutations of *CEBPA*

*Provisional entities*

AML with mutated *RUNX1*

AML with *BCR–ABL1*

**Therapy-related myeloid neoplasms**

**AML with myelodysplasia-related changes**

**AML, not otherwise specified (NOS)**

AML with minimal differentiation

AML without maturation

AML with maturation

Acute myelomonocytic leukemia

Acute monoblastic/monocytic leukemia

Pure erythroid leukemia

Acute megakaryoblastic leukemia

Acute basophilic leukemia

Acute panmyelosis with myelofibrosis

CONTINUED

TABLE 2.3 (CONTINUED)

**The World Health Organization 2016 classification of acute myeloid leukemia (AML) and related neoplasms***

**Myeloid sarcoma**

**Myeloid proliferations related to Down syndrome**

Transient abnormal myelopoiesis

Myeloid leukemia associated with Down syndrome

*Marrow blast count of ≥ 20% is required, except for AML with any of the recurrent genetic abnormalities: t(15;17), t(8;21), inv(16) or t(16;16).
Adapted from Arber et al., 2016.[3]

TABLE 2.4

**The 2017 European LeukemiaNet (ELN) risk stratification for acute myeloid leukemia based on genetic abnormalities***

| Risk category† | Genetic abnormality |
|---|---|
| Favorable | t(8;21)(q22;q22); *RUNX1–RUNX1T1* |
| | inv(16)(p13.1q22) or t(16;16)(p13.1;q22); *CBFB–MYH11* |
| | Mutated *NPM1* without *FLT3*-ITD or with *FLT3*-ITD$^{low}$ ‡ |
| | Bi-allelic mutated *CEBPA* |
| Intermediate | Mutated *NPM1* and *FLT3*-ITD$^{high}$ ‡ |
| | Wild type *NPM1* without *FLT3*-ITD or with *FLT3*-ITD$^{low}$ ‡ (without adverse-risk genetic lesions) |
| | t(9;11)(p21.3;q23.3); *MLLT3–KMT2A*§ |
| | Cytogenetic abnormalities not classified as favorable or adverse |

CONTINUED

TABLE 2.4 (CONTINUED)

**The 2017 European LeukemiaNet (ELN) risk stratification for acute myeloid leukemia based on genetic abnormalities***

| Risk category† | Genetic abnormality |
|---|---|
| Adverse | t(6;9)(p23;q34.1); *DEK–NUP214* |
| | t(v;11q23.3); *KMT2A* rearranged |
| | t(9;22)(q34.1;q11.2); *BCR–ABL1* |
| | inv(3)(q21.3q26.2) or t(3;3)(q21.3;q26.2); *GATA2, MECOM(EVI1)* |
| | –5 or del(5q); –7; –17/abn(17p) |
| | Complex karyotype,¶ monosomal karyotype** |
| | Wild type *NPM1* and *FLT3*-ITD$^{high}$ ‡ |
| | Mutated *RUNX1* †† |
| | Mutated *ASXL1* †† |
| | Mutated *TP53* ‡‡ |

*Excludes acute promyelocytic leukemia. Frequencies, response rates and outcome measures should be reported by risk category, and, if sufficient numbers are available, by specific genetic lesions indicated.
†The prognostic impact of a marker is treatment dependent and may change with new therapies.
‡ $^{Low}$, low allelic ratio (< 0.5); $^{high}$, high allelic ratio (≥ 0.5); semi-quantitative assessment of *FLT3*-ITD allelic ratio (using DNA fragment analysis) is determined from the ratio of the area under the curve for '*FLT3*-ITD' to '*FLT3*-wild type'; recent studies indicate that AML with *NPM1* mutation and *FLT3*-ITD low allelic ratio may also have a more favorable prognosis; therefore, these patients should not be routinely assigned to allogeneic hematopoietic cell transplantation.
§The presence of t(9;11)(p21.3;q23.3) takes precedence over rare concurrent adverse-risk gene mutations.
¶Three or more unrelated chromosome abnormalities in the absence of one of the World Health Organization-designated recurring translocations or inversions (i.e. t(8;21), inv(16) or t(16;16), t(9;11), t(v;11)(v;q23.3), t(6;9), inv(3) or t(3;3); AML with *BCR–ABL1*).
**Defined by the presence of a single monosomy (excluding loss of X or Y) in association with at least one additional monosomy or structural chromosome abnormality (excluding core-binding factor AML).
††These markers should not be used as an adverse prognostic marker if they co-occur with favorable-risk AML subtypes.
‡‡*TP53* mutations are significantly associated with AML with a complex and monosomal karyotype.
Adapted from Döhner et al., 2017.[4]

structural and/or numeric chromosomal abnormalities. Patients with t(15;17), for example, have an excellent prognosis (~85% cured), and those with t(8;21) or inv(16) (inversion of chromosome 16) also have a favorable prognosis (~55% cured), at least when treated appropriately (see 'Treatment' chapter). Patients with no cytogenetic abnormalities (cytogenetically normal AML; CN-AML) have an intermediate risk (~40% cured). Patients with a complex karyotype such as t(6;9), inv(3) or –7 (absence of chromosome 7) have an adverse prognosis, with few cures, particularly for older patients.

Cytogenetic analysis should be performed on the bone marrow aspirate taken at diagnosis in any patient suspected to have AML. The prognostic value of cytogenetic analysis is discussed in further detail in Chapter 5.

**Clinical genetic testing** for several mutated genes, particularly in patients with cytogenetically normal AML, can help with further risk stratification. Favorable genetic risk is observed in those with *NPM1* mutations without a high allelic ratio of *FLT3* internal tandem duplications (*FLT3*-ITD) and also in those with bi-allelic *CEBPA* mutations. Conversely, *TP53* mutations (typically, but not exclusively, observed in the setting of complex karyotypes) are associated with adverse risk. *IDH2* and *IDH1* mutations may contribute to prognostication but, more importantly, identify patients likely to respond to novel therapies that target these aberrant pathways, at least in the relapsed/refractory setting (see Chapter 3).

The number of genes mutated in AML that are known to have (or suspected of having) prognostic or therapeutic relevance is growing. Mutations beyond those used in the WHO and ELN systems are beyond the scope of this book; WHO is expected to add further genetic mutations in its 2018 update. Novel drugs that inhibit/modulate aberrant pathways activated by some of these genes (e.g. *IDH1*, *IDH2*, *KMT2A*) are currently being evaluated in clinical trials (see Chapter 6).

FLT3 is expressed on nearly all AML cells; the *FLT3* gene is mutated and constitutively activated in about 30% of patients with de novo AML.[5,6] The mutation is most commonly an ITD. *FLT3*-ITD is an adverse prognostic factor, associated with an increased risk for relapse and poor survival outcomes (see Chapter 5).[5,6] Furthermore, the ratio of mutated to wild-type alleles is an important consideration because a 'high' *FLT3*-ITD ratio (defined variably) confers greater risk; this allelic ratio is part of the updated ELN classification (see Table 2.4).[5,7] Mutations in the tyrosine kinase domain are less common (8% of patients) and have uncertain prognostic significance.[8,9] Identification of *FLT3*-ITD at diagnosis is important not only as a prognostic factor but also to identify patients who may respond to targeted treatments, such as a tyrosine kinase inhibitor (TKI); several TKIs in addition to midostaurin are being investigated in AML, including quizartinib, gilteritnib, crenolanib and sorafenib.

**Key points – diagnosis**

- Patients with acute myeloid leukemia (AML) typically present with vague symptoms resulting from pancytopenia. Fatigue, anorexia, weight loss and vague bone pain in the back or pelvis are common. Fever, infection or abnormal hemostasis may be the presenting symptom in some patients.
- Typical hematologic findings include normochromic, normocytic anemia, elevated white blood cell count and mild thrombocytopenia; the presence of Auer rods on light microscopy distinguishes acute myeloid from lymphoblastic leukemia.
- The diagnosis of AML is based on a finding of 20% or more myeloblasts although this is not a requirement in the presence of t(15;17), t(8;21), inv(16) or t(16;16) cytogenetic abnormalities.
- Cytogenetic and genetic tests are key aspects of the diagnostic work-up, required to aid rapid diagnosis, assess prognosis and inform treatment. Current genetic testing should include at least *FLT3* (with allelic ratio), *NPM1*, *CEBPA* (bi-allelic), *IDH1*, *IDH2* and *TP53*.
- The French–American–British morphologic classification of AML has been superseded by the World Health Organization classification and European LeukemiaNet stratification, which provide prognostic categories of 'favorable', 'intermediate' and 'adverse risk' based on cytogenetic and genetic findings.

## References


1. Kasper D, Fauci A, Hauser S et al. *Harrison's Principles of Internal Medicine*, 19th edn. McGraw-Hill, 2015.

2. Bennett JM, Catovsky D, Daniel MT et al. Proposals for the classification of the acute leukaemias. French-American-British (FAB) co-operative group. *Br J Haematol* 1976;33:451–8.

3. Arber DA, Orazi A, Hasserjian R et al. The 2016 revision to the World Health Organization classification of myeloid neoplasms and acute leukemia. *Blood* 2016;127:2391–405.

4. Döhner H, Estey E, Grimwade D et al. Diagnosis and management of AML in adults: 2017 ELN recommendations from an international expert panel. *Blood* 2017;129:424–47.

5. Whitman SP, Archer KJ, Feng L et al. Absence of the wild-type allele predicts poor prognosis in adult de novo acute myeloid leukemia with normal cytogenetics and the internal tandem duplication of FLT3: a cancer and leukemia group B study. *Cancer Res* 2001;61:7233–9.

6. Dohner H, Estey E, Grimwade D et al. Diagnosis and management of AML in adults: 2017 ELN recommendations from an international expert panel. *Blood* 2017;129:424–47.

7. Thiede C, Steudel C, Mohr B et al. Analysis of FLT3-activating mutations in 979 patients with acute myelogenous leukemia: association with FAB subtypes and identification of subgroups with poor prognosis. *Blood* 2002;99:4326–35.

8. Whitman SP, Ruppert AS, Radmacher MD et al. FLT3 D835/I836 mutations are associated with poor disease-free survival and a distinct gene-expression signature among younger adults with de novo cytogenetically normal acute myeloid leukemia lacking FLT3 internal tandem duplications. *Blood* 2008;111:1552–9.

9. Mead AJ, Linch DC, Hills RK et al. FLT3 tyrosine kinase domain mutations are biologically distinct from and have a significantly more favorable prognosis than FLT3 internal tandem duplications in patients with acute myeloid leukemia. *Blood* 2007;110:1262–70.

# 3 Treatment

Until relatively recently, a 'one way fits all' approach was used in the treatment of acute myeloid leukemia (AML). This chapter provides an overview of this standard therapeutic approach and illustrates the complexity of treatment decisions in weighing benefit versus risk in patients with different risk status. It also discusses novel approaches, including new targeted therapies that are emerging as our understanding of the genetic pathology of AML improves and the heterogeneity of the disease is recognized. Outcomes remain poor, highlighting the reality for AML patients that, when feasible, treatment on clinical trials remains the best option. The unique treatment of acute promyelocytic leukemia (APL) is considered separately at the end of this chapter.

## Standard treatment

The standard treatment course for patients with newly diagnosed AML is:

- induction chemotherapy to remove the majority of malignant cells and restore normal hematopoiesis, followed, once remission is achieved, by
- consolidation therapy with either high-dose non-myeloablative chemotherapy or allogeneic hematopoietic cell transplantation (alloHCT) to effectively eliminate residual disease.

## Standard induction chemotherapy

The regimen for standard induction chemotherapy was established from a series of studies conducted by the Cancer and Leukemia Group B in the 1970s and 1980s. It consists of daunorubicin for 3 days and cytosine arabinoside (cytarabine; AraC), 100–200 mg/m$^2$ per day, administered as a continuous infusion for 7 days, commonly known as the 3+7 schedule.[1] It is recognized today that previously used doses of daunorubicin 45 mg/m$^2$/day were suboptimal; a dose intensity of daunorubicin 60–90 mg/m$^2$ is now the norm.

The aim of induction chemotherapy is complete remission (CR), defined morphologically as fewer than 5% blasts on a bone marrow aspirate, with recovery of blood counts to normal (hemoglobin > 110 g/L, absolute neutrophil count >1000/mm$^3$ *and* platelet count >100000/mm$^3$). CR is achieved 4–5 weeks after initiating induction chemotherapy in 60–70% of patients. However, all patients require some form of consolidation therapy following achievement of CR to prevent disease recurrence. The definition of CR is further defined based on the detection of residual disease by cytogenetic or molecular testing. Treatment for patients who do not achieve CR after at least two cycles of induction chemotherapy (refractory or relapsed disease) is discussed on page 45.

Mortality due to complications after induction chemotherapy – largely due to infection – varies from 3% to 15% and is related to performance status (PS), age, leukemic complications at presentation and medical comorbidities.[2] PS refers to the general medical condition of the patient and is scored from 0 to 5, where PS 0 denotes a fully active patient and PS 4 denotes a completely disabled patient who is confined to bed/chair (PS 5 is dead). Assessment of organ function, medical comorbidities, PS and other disease- or patient-specific factors helps to determine patient 'fitness' for intensive therapy, but the final decision on eligibility remains largely subjective.

**Use of alternative anthracyclines.** While daunorubicin has been the most commonly used anthracycline in the management of AML, alternatives have been considered. Idarubicin has a potentially superior pharmacokinetic profile to daunorubicin. Comparisons of these two agents in four large trials showed a significant improvement in CR rates with idarubicin, but disease-free survival (DFS) improved in only one trial. Another large trial conducted by the French GOELAM group found no benefit with idarubicin in terms of inducing remission or long-term survival. Successive Eastern Cooperative Oncology Group studies demonstrated that daunorubicin 60 mg/m$^2$ and idarubicin 12 mg/m$^2$ had equivalent response rates (reviewed in Cassileth et al.[1]). There was some suggestion that increasing the dose of daunorubicin to 90 mg/m$^2$ would improve outcomes;[3] however, current opinion is that daunorubicin 60 mg/m$^2$/day for 3 days is optimal, based on the balance between efficacy and toxicity.[4,5]

**High-dose AraC for induction.** Several studies have explored the use of high-dose AraC (six doses of AraC 2–3 g/m$^2$ at 12-hour intervals) in induction chemotherapy. While a few earlier studies suggested a benefit,[6,7] more recent data, including the SWOG S1203 randomized controlled trial, showed no benefit of high-dose AraC (with or without vorinostat) over a conventional-dose 3+7 induction regimen.[8]

## Newly approved drugs

After more than three decades with virtually no new agents, four new treatments were recently approved (Table 3.1). Midostaurin and enasidenib in particular highlight the value and potential for genetic testing in AML. Below are summarized new agents for initial therapy: midostaurin, CPX-351, and gemtuzumab ozogamicin. Enasidenib is discussed under the treatment of relapsed disease on page 47.

***Midostaurin*** is an oral multiple tyrosine kinase inhibitor (TKI) that mainly inhibits FLT3 but also PDGFR, KIT and other tyrosine kinases. Midostaurin was approved by the US Food and Drug Administration (FDA) in April 2017 for use in combination with standard intensive chemotherapy in the first-line treatment of adults with *FLT3*-mutated AML; the US label specifies use of the LeukoStrat CDx *FLT3* Mutation Assay to detect the *FLT3* mutation. Early clinical trials with midostaurin as monotherapy showed only modest clinical benefit, but this was considered worthy of future research given the poor prognosis of patients with *FLT3*-mutated AML. Laboratory studies of midostaurin in combination with chemotherapy demonstrated a synergistic effect, and clinical studies demonstrated that the combination was safe and promising.[9] The RATIFY trial was an international, randomized, placebo-controlled trial of midostaurin, 50 mg twice daily for 2 weeks, starting after completion of chemotherapy, in adults (aged 18–60 years) with newly diagnosed AML.[10] Chemotherapy was daunorubicin (60 g/m$^2$) and AraC in a standard 3+7 schedule. A total of 717 patients were randomized, 77% of whom had a *FLT3* internal tandem duplication (*FLT3*-ITD); patients with a *FLT3* tyrosine kinase domain (*FLT3*-TKD) were also eligible. Overall survival (OS) was longer in the midostaurin-treated patients (hazard ratio [HR] 0.78, $p = 0.009$), as was event-free survival (HR 0.78, $p = 0.002$) (Figure 3.1). Notably, these survival data held up after censoring for transplant, and the benefit of

TABLE 3.1

**New drugs approved for the treatment of AML in 2017**

| Drug (brand name; manufacturer) | Mechanism of action | Date of FDA approval | Indication |
|---|---|---|---|
| Midostaurin (Rydapt; Novartis) | Inhibits FLT3 (plus PDGFR, KIT and other tyrosine kinases) | April 2017* | Newly diagnosed *FLT3*-positive AML,‡ in combination with standard cytarabine and daunorubicin induction and cytarabine consolidation |
| Enasidenib (Idhifa; Celgene) | Oral inhibitor of IDH2, which catalyzes the conversion of isocitrate to alpha-ketoglutarate in the Krebs cycle | August 2017 | Relapsed or refractory AML with *IDH2* mutation‡ |
| CPX-351 (Vyxeos; Jazz Pharmaceuticals) | Cytarabine plus daunorubicin in a liposomal formulation for injection | August 2017 | Newly diagnosed therapy-related AML or AML with myelodysplasia-related changes |
| Gemtuzumab ozogamicin (Mylotarg; Pfizer) | Anti-CD33 monoclonal antibody drug conjugate (antibody–calicheamicin) | Sept 2017† | Adults with newly diagnosed CD33-positive AML<br>Patients aged ≥ 2 years with relapsed or refractory CD33-positive AML |

* Approved by the European Medicines Agency (EMA), September 2017. †Positive opinion from the EMA Committee for Human Medicinal Products received February 2018. ‡As detected by an FDA-approved test.

AML, acute myeloid leukemia; FDA, Food and Drug Administration; IDH, isocitrate dehydrogenase; PDGFR platelet-derived growth factor receptor.

midostaurin was seen across all *FLT3* mutation groups (ITD allelic ratio high or low, and *FLT3*-TKD mutation).

***CPX-351*** (Vyxeos) is a combination of two standard chemotherapy agents, AraC and daunorubicin, in a synergistic 5:1 molar ratio, encapsulated in nanoscale liposomes; this is expected to optimize the delivery and antileukemic effects of the individual agents. Early trials suggested efficacy in a particularly poor-risk subset of patients with therapy-related AML or AML with myelodysplasia-related changes. In the Phase III trial, 309 patients aged 60–75 years were randomized to receive CPX-351 or conventional chemotherapy with daunorubicin plus cytarabine (3+7 schedule).[11] Median OS was 9.6 months with CPX-351, versus 6 months with standard chemotherapy (HR 0.69; $p$ = 0.005). This survival benefit is clinically meaningful: at 2 years, 31% of patients enrolled in the CPX-351 arm of the study remained alive, compared with 12% in the 3+7 arm. CPX-351 was approved by the FDA in August 2017 for adults with newly diagnosed therapy-related AML or AML with myelodysplasia-related changes.

***Gemtuzumab ozogamicin (GO)*** is an antibody–toxin (chalicheamicin) conjugate that targets CD33+ myeloblasts. It was first approved by the FDA in 2000 but was later withdrawn from the market because of safety concerns (particularly hepatotoxicity/veno-occlusive disease). However, clinical trials continued and the safety concerns were overcome. Further studies explored GO at a lower dose and with fractionated administration, alone and in combination with chemotherapy. GO was approved by the FDA in 2017 for use in combination with chemotherapy for the first-line treatment of adults with AML, based primarily on the results of the ALFA-0701 trial, the results of which were published in 2012 and then updated in 2014.[12,13] In ALFA-0701, low-dose fractionated GO (3 mg/m$^2$ on days 1, 4 and 7) was administered in combination with daunorubicin (60 mg/m$^2$) and AraC given in a typical 3+7 schedule. (The previously approved dosage of GO in 2000 was 9 mg/m$^2$ on days 1 and 14, as monotherapy, or 6 mg/m$^2$ as a single dose in combination with chemotherapy [SWOG 0106], which proved too toxic.[14]) Long-term follow-up results of the ALFA trial demonstrated a marked event-free survival benefit with GO: 3-year event-free survival was 31%, compared with 19% in the control group (HR 0.66, $p$ = 0.0026), although OS was not significantly improved (3-year OS 44% vs 36%). The treatment effect appears to be

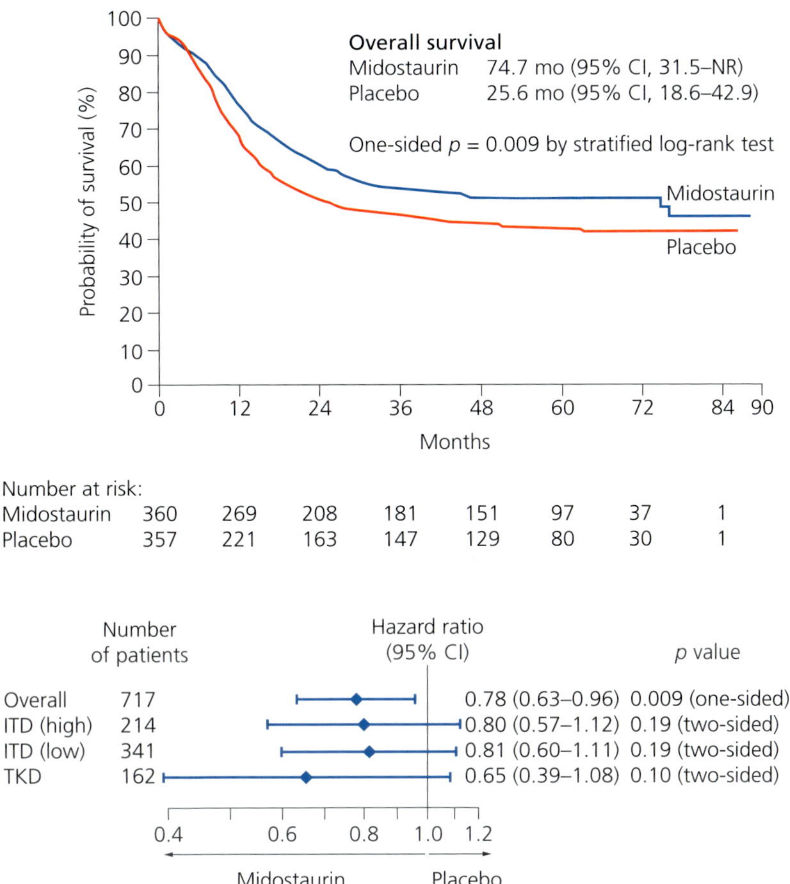


**Figure 3.1** Overall survival (OS) with midostaurin in patients with newly diagnosed AML in the RATIFY trial. (a) Kaplan–Meier curves for median OS; tick marks indicate censoring of data. (b) Between-group comparison of OS with stratification according to subtype of *FLT3* mutation: point mutation in the tyrosine kinase domain (TKD) or internal tandem duplication (ITD) with either a high (> 0.7) or low (0.05–0.7) ratio of mutated to wild-type alleles. CI, confidence interval; mo, months; NR, not reached. Reproduced with permission from Stone et al., 2017.[10]

seen in patients with more favorable risk. Additional evidence of efficacy with low-dose GO plus chemotherapy had also been observed in mostly younger, favorable-risk patients, as previously reported by the Medical Research Council AML15 study (GO at 3 mg/m$^2$ given during courses 1 and 3).[15]

Clinical trials with GO in a different patient population were also successful. The AML-19 study in 237 older patients (> 60 years) who were unfit for chemotherapy showed that fractionated lower-dose GO monotherapy (6 mg/m$^2$ on day 1; 3 mg/m$^2$ on day 8) was superior to best supportive care (BSC).[16] Maintenance therapy was permitted in the GO arm at 2 mg/m$^2$ monthly. Median OS was 4.9 months with GO and 3.6 months with BSC (HR 0.69; 95% confidence interval [CI] 0.53–0.90; $p = 0.005$); The 1-year OS rate was 24.3% with GO and 9.7% with BSC. Survival benefit was observed in subsets of patients with favorable- and intermediate-risk cytogenetics but not in those with adverse-risk cytogenetics.

## Standard consolidation therapy (following intensive induction)

Patients are estimated to have $10^{12}$ leukemic cells at diagnosis, which intensive induction chemotherapy reduces by 4–5 orders of magnitude (logs). While this effectively reduces the disease burden by 99.9%, $10^7$–$10^8$ residual leukemic cells still remain. Detectable residual cells are referred to as measurable residual disease (MRD; formerly minimal residual disease). These residual cells are substantially diluted by the normal cell population, such that they can only be measured by sensitive techniques such as multiparameter flow cytometry or real-time polymerase chain reaction assays; they cannot be detected by morphology alone.

It is important to recognize from the outset that outcomes after remission is achieved (termed DFS) in young adults (< 60 years) have improved steadily over the last three decades: 5-year DFS has improved from 11% to 37%. However, the prognosis for older patients (> 60 years) remains dismal (5-year DFS has improved from 6% to 12%).[17]

Consolidation therapy is required once CR is achieved with induction chemotherapy, in order to eliminate all residual disease; disease recurrence is inevitable without this treatment (Table 3.2). For patients who achieve first CR (CR1) following intensive induction chemotherapy, the options for consolidation therapy are:

- intensive high-dose (non-myeloablative) chemotherapy
- allogeneic hematopoietic cell transplantation (alloHCT)
- autologous HCT (autoHCT).

**Intensive (non-myeloablative) consolidation chemotherapy.** Repeated courses of high-dose AraC (usually three or four at monthly intervals) – alone or in combination with other drugs – has been found to be effective as consolidation therapy in the treatment of AML, particularly in the favorable-risk subset.[18,19] The conventional dose for high-dose AraC has been 3000 mg/m$^2$; however, emerging data suggest that this dose provides no advantage over intermediate doses of 1000–1500 mg/m$^2$.[5] The consensus is that the intermediate dose of AraC needs to be administered for 3–4 cycles, and there appears to be little benefit in combining this with additional chemotherapy.[5] It is important to note that younger favorable-risk patients have worse outcomes when doses below 1000 mg/m$^2$ are used for consolidation.[8] Many physicians, however, still prefer higher doses of AraC at least for younger, favorable-risk patients. Guidelines for dosing of consolidation chemotherapy are provided by European LeukemiaNet.[5]

**Allogeneic hematopoietic cell transplantation** involves the infusion of hematopoietic stem cells from a related or unrelated donor (following a conditioning regimen), to induce a graft-versus-leukemia effect in order to eliminate residual disease. AlloHCT is the best option in terms of reducing the risk of relapse (Table 3.3) although the benefit is somewhat offset by increased treatment-related mortality (TRM) due

TABLE 3.2

**Probability of survival and relapse with consolidation therapy according to cytogenetic risk**

| | Good risk | Intermediate risk | High risk |
|---|---|---|---|
| Probability of relapse | 25% | 50% | > 70% |
| 4-year probability of survival | > 60% | 40–50% | < 20% |

Data from Lowenberg et al. 2003.[20]

to complications, including graft-versus-host disease. Large prospective trials have consistently shown that alloHCT with a standard myeloablative conditioning regimen is the most effective treatment for patients with AML at CR1, with a relapse risk of 24–36% (compared with 46–61% with autoHCT or chemotherapy). Whilst none of these trials individually showed a benefit in terms of OS, mainly because of the high TRM (10–25%), a meta-analysis demonstrated significant OS benefit for adverse-risk AML (HR 0.73; 95% CI 0.59–0.90) and intermediate-risk AML (HR 0.83; 95% CI 0.74–0.93) but not for favorable-risk AML (HR 1.07; 95% CI 0.83–1.38).[21]

AlloHCT should not be used initially for patients in the favorable-risk cytogenetic group as these patients respond well to consolidation with conventional non-myeloablative chemotherapy. However, it can be considered for patients in this group if their disease relapses and after a second CR is achieved.

In the intermediate- and adverse-risk groups (collectively referred to as unfavorable risk), the TRM associated with alloHCT may be acceptable in the context of improving DFS and OS, given the reduction in risk of relapse observed with alloHCT. An intergroup study in patients with unfavorable-risk AML at CR1 reported a 5-year OS rate of 44%, compared with 15% with chemotherapy or autoHCT[22]; a similar but less dramatic difference was reported in the AML-10 trial.[23] However, two other studies failed to show an advantage of alloHCT over chemotherapy or autoHCT. In all the studies, the outcome with chemotherapy or autoHCT alone was dismal.

TABLE 3.3

**Relapse risk with allogeneic HCT, autologous HCT and chemotherapy in Phase III trials**

| Study | Allogeneic HCT | Autologous HCT | Chemotherapy |
|---|---|---|---|
| GIMMEMA[24] | 24 | 40 | 57 |
| GOELAM[25] | 28 | 45 | 55 |
| MRC[23] | 19 | 35 | 53 |
| ECOG/SWOG[1] | 29 | 48 | 61 |

Values are relapse risk (%).
HCT, hematopoietic cell transplantation.

Based on the available data, it is reasonable to proceed with human leukcocyte antigen (HLA)-identical alloHCT in patients at CR1 who have intermediate- or adverse-risk disease, if a donor is available. That said, data from most large prospective clinical trials did not show any improvement in OS after alloHCT in CR1 in the intermediate-risk group, although one study reported a significant improvement in DFS. Thus, there is no consensus on the use of alloHCT in CR1 for the intermediate-risk group, and the optimal therapeutic strategy for these patients is still evolving. If an HLA-identical donor is available, other parameters can be used to guide the decision-making process. Factors that favor alloHCT in CR1 are shown in Table 3.4. Experts suggest that if the risk of relapse is greater than 30%, alloHCT is justified to decrease this risk, offsetting the risk of TRM associated with the procedure.[5] Increasingly, patients without HLA-identical donors benefit from alloHCT using alternative techniques such as haploidentical donors with T-cell depletion, or umbilical cord blood transplantation. Furthermore, TRM rates may be improved with the administration of reduced-intensity conditioning (RIC) regimens, at least in patients with medical comorbidities that are associated with high TRM using conventional myeloablative conditioning. Expanded use of RIC for older AML patients may improve access to HCT and improve outcomes for this particularly high-risk subset.[26]

Notably, the outcomes with alloHCT are profoundly affected by disease burden at the time of the procedure. Patients with active leukemia, or even those in morphologic remission but with MRD, fare poorly, with high relapse rates.[27,28]

***Role of consolidation chemotherapy before alloHCT.*** Retrospective analysis of data from the International Bone Marrow Transplant Registry (IBMTR) and European Group for Blood and Marrow Transplantation (EBMT) suggests that consolidation chemotherapy before alloHCT does not benefit patients with AML in CR1. Another retrospective analysis from a single center showed similar findings and suggested that multiple courses of chemotherapy before alloHCT had a deleterious effect.

***Bone marrow versus peripheral blood stem cells.*** Retrospective analysis of the EBMT and IBMTR data showed that use of peripheral blood stem cells (PBSC) is beneficial in patients with advanced AML but not for those in CR1, although another retrospective study did

TABLE 3.4

**Factors that influence the success of allogeneic hematopoietic cell transplantation following CR1**

| Favorable factors | Unfavorable factors |
|---|---|
| Age (< 40 years) | High white blood cell count at diagnosis (> 30 000–40 000/mm³), which is associated with a high risk of relapse |
| | > 1 cycle of chemotherapy to achieve CR1 |
| | Available HLA-identical donor |
| | Presence of MRD after induction therapy |
| | Molecular markers (see page 26) |

CR1, first complete remission; HLA, human leukocyte antigen; MRD, measurable residual disease

show a benefit for patients with AML in CR1 who underwent PBSC transplantation. A more recent retrospective analysis of the Acute Leukemia Working Party/EBMT registry data suggests that the use of bone marrow improves outcomes compared with PBSC transplantation when the dose of bone marrow CD34+ cells exceeded $2.7 \times 10^6$. The only prospective study to address this issue demonstrated earlier engraftment, reduced TRM and improved DFS with PBSC transplantation, but there was no difference in OS.[29] Use of bone marrow is associated with a lower risk of chronic graft-versus-host disease.

**Autologous hematopoietic cell transplantation** involves re-infusing the patient's own stem cells following induction therapy, and can be understood best as high-dose chemotherapy with stem-cell rescue. AutoHCT for patients in CR1 has largely fallen out of practice in the USA, although it may still provide a reasonable option for selected patients.

## Treatment selection

Decisions about the treatment course for individual patients are strongly influenced by cytogenetic risk, together with additional parameters such as age, comorbidities at diagnosis, white blood cell count at diagnosis, response to induction chemotherapy, and type of consolidation therapy.

- In the favorable-risk group, alloHCT is generally not considered in view of a TRM of 10–20%, whereas repeated cycles of high-dose non-myeloablative consolidation chemotherapy can achieve long-term DFS rates above 60%, with TRM rates below 5% (at least in younger patients).
- In the adverse-risk group, the choice would be to proceed with alloHCT in CR1 where possible, given the well-recognized dismal outcome with chemotherapy (Figure 3.2).
- In the intermediate-risk group, which constitutes 40–50% of patients with AML, the options in CR1 are less clearly defined. This group is heterogeneous in their response to therapy and most have a normal karyotype. New markers and MRD assessment could help identify subsets at high risk of relapse and therefore candidates for HCT. There is no clear indication for autoHCT in CR1, although it may be beneficial for patients who are ineligible for repeated consolidation chemotherapy or alloHCT.

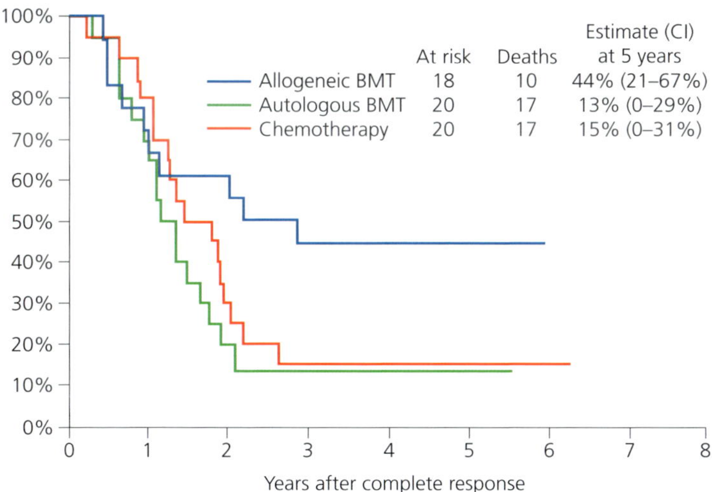


**Figure 3.2** Estimated survival distribution with patients with unfavorable-risk acute myeloid leukemia. BMT, bone marrow transplantation; CI, confidence interval. Adapted from Slovak et al., 2000[34]

Depending on the risk status at diagnosis, both approaches to consolidation (non-myeloablative chemotherapy or HCT) are potentially curative. In consolidation, intensive chemotherapy is associated with the lowest TRM but the highest risk of disease relapse, whereas alloHCT is associated with the lowest risk of disease recurrence but has a relatively higher risk of TRM.[30] AutoHCT has an intermediate risk of TRM, and most prospective trials have demonstrated a reduction in relapse rate compared with chemotherapy alone. The choice of consolidation therapy is strongly influenced by the cytogenetic risk group, which influences the risk of relapse and probability of survival (see Table 3.2).

## Induction in older and physically 'unfit' patients

Lower-intensity therapies such as the hypomethylating agents (decitabine, azacitidine) and low-dose AraC may have a role in subsets of patients, particularly those who are physically 'unfit' for intensive therapy, and older patients with adverse-risk disease who are unlikely to benefit from intensive treatments. With such therapies, three or four cycles of treatment may be required before a response is seen, and therapy may be reasonably continued indefinitely for responding patients if there is no disease progression. Clearly, outcomes with all such treatments remain very poor; clinical trials should be recommended. Of note, ongoing clinical trials with azacitidine and the Bcl-2 protein inhibitor venetoclax have shown encouraging results; the approach is now in phase III trials.

## Treatment of relapsed and refractory disease

Induction chemotherapy fails to induce remission in a proportion of patients. By convention, a patient is stated to have primary refractory AML if hematologic remission has not been achieved despite at least two cycles of induction chemotherapy. The prognosis of these patients remains poor despite salvage chemotherapy and alloHCT. AlloHCT for patients not in remission may be considered for younger, fit patients with primary refractory AML

**Intensive salvage chemotherapy and allogeneic hematopoietic cell transplantation.** Overall consensus is that patients with relapsed or refractory disease should receive alloHCT as part of consolidation following successful re-induction with salvage chemotherapy. Unfortunately, the proportion of patients with relapsed and refractory disease who achieve CR is less than 50%, and fewer than 30% actually proceed to alloHCT.[5,31]

The optimal salvage regimen has yet to be defined, and where possible, patients should be encouraged to enroll on a clinical trial. A commonly used salvage regimen is a combination of fludarabine, high-dose cytosine and idarubicin (FLAG-IDA regimen). Even for patients who do not achieve remission, there is a potential role for alloHCT, and one approach has been to use a combination of fludarabine, high-dose cytosine and amsacrine and then proceed with alloHCT at peak cytopenia, which occurs 10–15 days after initiating salvage chemotherapy. With this approach, CR rates of 70–90% and long-term survival of 30–45% have been reported.[5,32]

Factors that predict poor response rates and poor long-term survival in this cohort of patients include: short duration of CR1 in the case of relapsed disease, complex and high-risk karyotype, increasing age and history of prior alloHCT.[37] Data from the Center for International Bone Marrow Transplant Registry suggest that, for patients whose disease relapses after alloHCT, 3-year survival rates were 4%, 12%, 26% and 38% for relapses that happened within 1–6 months, 6–24 months, 2–3 years and more than 3 years after first alloHCT, respectively.[5,32]

## New treatment options for patients with relapsed or refractory disease

For patients with relapsed disease who are not fit to receive intensive salvage chemotherapy and alloHCT, treatment with hypomethylating agents can be considered, though response rates are usually less than 20% and the duration of response is only a few months in the majority of those who do respond.[5]

**Enasidenib** is an oral inhibitor of isocitrate dehydrogenase 2 (IDH2) recently approved by FDA for relapsed or refractory AML with *IDH2* mutation. IDH2 is an enzyme that catalyzes the conversion of isocitrate to α-ketoglutarate in the Krebs cycle (Figure 3.3). Mutations in the genes that encode mitochondrial IDH2 (and cytosolic IDH1) ultimately lead to aberrations in the Krebs cycle that result in the production of 2-hydroxyglutarate (2HG), which has been shown to act

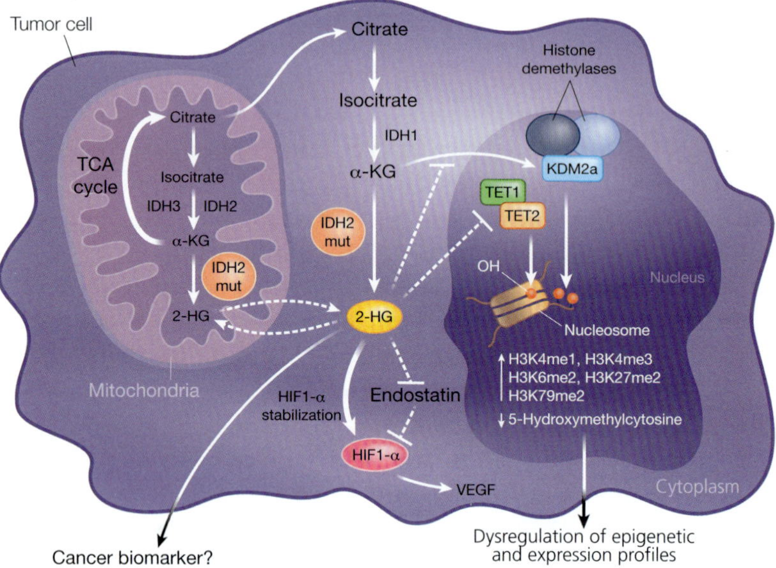


**Figure 3.3** The Krebs cycle. Enasidenib inhibits aberrant isocitrate dehydrogenase 2 (IDH2mut), preventing accumulation of the oncometabolite 2-hydroxyglutarate (2HG). 2HG results in aberrant nucleosome activity and epigenetic changes. Reproduced with permission from Presner & Chinnaiyan, 2011.[8]

as a so-called 'oncometabolite'. Increased levels of 2HG result in increased DNA methylation and chromatin modifications that affect gene expression and contribute to oncogenesis in several different cancers, including AML.[34–36] In early studies in AML, enasidenib reduced 2HG levels by more than 90% and reversed these aberrant epigenetic changes, resulting in myeloid cell differentiation.[37–40] *IDH2* mutations occur in approximately 12% of patients with AML, particularly in older adults with a normal karyotype.[38,41]

Enasidenib was evaluated in a Phase I/II first-in-human trial involving 199 patients with relapsed or refractory AML and the *IDH2* mutation.[38] The drug, given once daily, was well tolerated, allowing it to be administered largely in the outpatient setting. The FDA press release noted that 19% of patients treated for at least 6 months achieved a CR that lasted a median of 8.2 months. Moreover, patients who did not achieve objective CR also benefited, with reduced transfusion needs and stable disease for a median of 9.6 months. Furthermore, 34 of 157 patients who required blood or platelet transfusions at the start of the study no longer required transfusions after treatment.[38,42] The overall response rate was 40% (including 19% CR), with a median response duration of 5.8 months and a median OS of 9.3 months. Median OS was 19.7 months in patients who achieved CR. These results supported rapid approval of enasidenib by the FDA, for the treatment of adults with relapsed or refractory *IDH2*-mutated AML.[38] Ongoing studies are combining enasidenib with chemotherapy in the first-line treatment of AML.

**Ivosidenib.** In AML, mutations in *IDH1* occur slightly less frequently than in *IDH2* and may also be targeted by similar compounds. Ivosidenib (AG-120), an oral selective inhibitor of *IDH1*, is likely to be approved by the FDA in the near future for relapsed and refractory *IDH1*-mutated AML, given similar clinical results.[43]

**Gemtuzumab ozogamicin** (see page 38) was approved by the FDA in 2017 as monotherapy in patients ≥ 2 years of age with relapsed or refractory AML. A Phase II single-arm study (MyloFrance-1) demonstrated activity of GO as monotherapy in the relapsed/refractory setting, with a CR rate of 26% (95% CI 16–40%) and relapse-free survival of 11.6 months.[44] Patients received 3 mg/m$^2$ GO monotherapy on days 1, 4 and 7.

## Treatment of acute promyelocytic leukemia

Patients with APL have an excellent prognosis; greater than 85% of patients are cured. With initial therapy, nearly all patients with APL who survive induction go on to achieve remission. However, the frequency of early death is higher in APL than in other AML subtypes due to the risk of fatal hemorrhage, especially in patients presenting with a high leukocyte count (> 10 000/uL).

Available treatments for APL include all-*trans*-retinoic acid (ATRA) with either chemotherapy or arsenic trioxide (ATO). An important component of APL therapy is the use of oral ATRA therapy; ATRA induces differentiation of malignant promyelocytes, thus reducing disseminated intravascular coagulation (DIC) very effectively over 3–4 days. Initiation of ATRA at suspicion of APL based on morphologic and clinical grounds, before molecular or cytogenetic confirmation of the *PML–RARA* fusion, reduces early fatal hemorrhage in these patients.

Use of ATRA is also associated with the development of 'APL syndrome' (formerly ATRA syndrome or differentiation syndrome) in the first weeks of treatment. It is characterized by fever, fluid retention, dyspnea, pulmonary infiltrates, pleural and pericardial effusion, and hypoxemia. Patients with APL syndrome typically have rising white blood cell count due to ATRA- or ATO-induced differentiation of malignant promyelocytes. Glucocorticoids, chemotherapy (to reduce leukocyte count) and supportive measures are indicated for management of the syndrome. Temporary discontinuation of ATRA is necessary in severe cases (i.e. respiratory distress and renal failure).

ATRA monotherapy has a high response rate, but also a high relapse rate; the addition of conventional chemotherapy to ATRA was the standard of care for all APL patients until 2013, when novel therapy for low-risk APL was definitively shown to be superior to ATRA plus chemotherapy in a randomized trial.[45] ATRA (45 mg/m$^2$/day) plus ATO (0.15 mg/kg/day) was compared with ATRA plus idarubicin in patients with low-risk APL (low leukocyte count at presentation), . ATRA/ATO was superior to ATRA/idarubicin and is now the standard of care for such patients. CR rates in low-risk disease approach 100%, with excellent long-term survival. Patients with high-risk APL (due to high leukocyte count) were not included in this study. Such patients require immediate cytoreduction because of a high frequency of life-threatening APL syndrome, often with rapidly rising leukocyte count, after initiation of ATRA. High-risk patients are at increased risk for death during induction because of this syndrome, as well as increased frequency of hemorrhagic complications (related to DIC).

Options for treatment of patients with high-risk APL are many, and are typically chemotherapy plus ATRA, as was previously used in all patients,[46–50] although some clinical trials also demonstrate activity of ATRA/ATO plus gemtuzumab ozogamicin.[46–50]

For patients treated with ATRA and chemotherapy, ATO may be incorporated into post-remission therapy to reduce relapse and/or toxicity, especially for high-risk patients.[49,51] ATO monotherapy for induction is effective and has been studied in areas of the developing world without access to ATRA.[52]

In high-risk patients, sequential monitoring for the PML–RARA gene during CR1 is considered standard. As the risk of relapse in low-risk APL is quite low, MRD testing in CR1 may not be necessary in this subset. Fortunately, relapsing APL responds well to ATO-based therapy[53] and may be cured with ATO or transplantation (notably autoHCT for patients who are MRD negative in second CR).

**Key points – treatment options**

- Historically, treatment of acute myeloid leukemia (AML) adopted a 'one way fits all' approach, using induction chemotherapy to kill large numbers of leukemic cells. In individualized consolidation therapy, the same effect is achieved with either repeated intensive non-myeloablative chemotherapy or, for eligible patients, allogeneic or autologous hematopoietic cell transplantation.
- Treatment is strongly influenced by a patient's cytogenetic/molecular risk profile, and is informed by other factors, such as age, fitness and the response to induction chemotherapy; it is therefore highly individualized.
- Whilst the outlook for younger adults (< 60 years) has gradually improved over recent years, the outlook for older patients remains dismal.
- Acute promyelocytic leukemia (APL) therapy has high cure rates but early death rates remain an issue for patients presenting with a high white blood cell count.
- Midostaurin inhibits several tyrosine kinases, including FLT3, which is constitutively activated in about 30% of patients with AML, usually because of an internal tandem duplication (*FLT3*-ITD). It is indicated for use in combination with standard induction chemotherapy for the first-line treatment of adults with *FLT3*-ITD.
- Enasidenib inhibits aberrant isocitrate dehydrogenase 2 (IDH2) which catalyzes formation of the oncometabolite 2-hydroxyglutarate. *IDH2* mutations occur in approximately 12% of AML patients, particularly in older adults with normal karyotype. Enasidenib is approved for the treatment of relapsed or refractory AML with the *IDH2* mutation.

- The anti-CD33 monoclonal antibody–drug conjugate gemtuzumab ozogamicin has been approved for first-line treatment of AML, following modifications to the dosage and schedule in order to address the safety concerns that arose following its initial approval. It is also approved for relapsed AML (including in pediatric patients); both indications are with a reduced fractionated dose schedule.
- Clinical trials focusing on small, genetically similar subsets are becoming the norm; success with molecular targeted therapies approved in 2017 is likely to herald a shift towards a more targeted, individualized approach.
- All patients with relapsed or refractory disease should be considered for allogeneic hematopoietic cell transplantation.

## References


1. Cassileth PA, Harrington DP, Appelbaum FR et al. Chemotherapy compared with autologous or allogeneic bone marrow transplantation in the management of acute myeloid leukemia in first remission. *N Engl J Med* 1998;339:1649–56.

2. Philip C, George B, Ganapule A et al. Acute myeloid leukaemia: challenges and real world data from India. *Br J Haematol* 2015;170: 110–17.

3. Fernandez HF, Sun Z, Yao X et al. Anthracycline dose intensification in acute myeloid leukemia. *N Engl J Med* 2009;361:1249–59.

4. Burnett AK, Russell NH, Hills RK et al. A randomized comparison of daunorubicin 90 mg/m$^2$ vs 60 mg/m$^2$ in AML induction: results from the UK NCRI AML17 trial in 1206 patients. *Blood* 2015;125:3878–85.

5. Dohner H, Estey E, Grimwade D et al. Diagnosis and management of AML in adults: 2017 ELN recommendations from an international expert panel. *Blood* 2017;129:424–47.

6. Bishop JF, Matthews JP, Young GA et al. A randomized study of high-dose cytarabine in induction in acute myeloid leukemia. *Blood* 1996;87:1710–17.

7. Weick JK, Kopecky KJ, Appelbaum FR et al. A randomized investigation of high-dose versus standard-dose cytosine arabinoside with daunorubicin in patients with previously untreated acute myeloid leukemia: a Southwest Oncology Group study. *Blood* 1996;88:2841–51.

8. Garcia-Manero G, Othus M, Pagel J et al. A randomized phase III study of standard cytarabine plus daunorubicin (7+3) therapy versus idarubicin with high dose cytarabine (IA) with or without vorinostat (IA+V) in younger patients with previously untreated acute myeloid leukemia (AML). *Blood* 2016;128:901.

9. Stone RM, Fischer T, Paquette R et al. Phase IB study of the FLT3 kinase inhibitor midostaurin with chemotherapy in younger newly diagnosed adult patients with acute myeloid leukemia. *Leukemia* 2012;26:2061–8.

10. Stone RM, Mandrekar SJ, Sanford BL et al. Midostaurin plus chemotherapy for acute myeloid leukemia with a FLT3 mutation. *N Engl J Med* 2017;377:454–64.

11. Lancet J, Uy G, Cortes J et al. Final results of a phase III randomized trial of CPX-351 versus 7+3 in older patients with newly diagnosed high risk (secondary) AML. *J Clin Oncol* 2016;34 (suppl):abstr 7000.

12. Castaigne S, Pautas C, Terre C et al. Effect of gemtuzumab ozogamicin on survival of adult patients with de-novo acute myeloid leukaemia (ALFA-0701): a randomised, open-label, phase 3 study. *Lancet* 2012;379:1508–16.

13. Castaigne S, Pautas C, Terré C et al. Final analysis of the ALFA 0701 study. *Blood* 2014;124.

14. Petersdorf SH, Kopecky KJ, Slovak M et al. A phase 3 study of gemtuzumab ozogamicin during induction and postconsolidation therapy in younger patients with acute myeloid leukemia. *Blood* 2013;121:4854–60.

15. Burnett AK, Hills RK, Milligan D et al. Identification of patients with acute myeloblastic leukemia who benefit from the addition of gemtuzumab ozogamicin: results of the MRC AML15 trial. *J Clin Oncol* 2011;29:369–77.

16. Amadori S, Suciu S, Selleslag D et al. Gemtuzumab ozogamicin versus best supportive care in older patients with newly diagnosed acute myeloid leukemia unsuitable for intensive chemotherapy: results of the randomized phase III EORTC-GIMEMA AML-19 trial. *J Clin Oncol* 2016;34:972–9.

17. Appelbaum FR, Rowe JM, Radich J, Dick JE. Acute myeloid leukemia. *Hematology Am Soc Hematol Educ Program* 2001:62–86.

18. Byrd JC, Dodge RK, Carroll A et al. Patients with t(8;21)(q22;q22) and acute myeloid leukemia have superior failure-free and overall survival when repetitive cycles of high-dose cytarabine are administered. *J Clin Oncol* 1999;17:3767–75.

19. Byrd JC, Ruppert AS, Mrozek K et al. Repetitive cycles of high-dose cytarabine benefit patients with acute myeloid leukemia and inv(16)(p13q22) or t(16;16)(p13;q22): results from CALGB 8461. *J Clin Oncol* 2004;22:1087–94.

20. Lowenberg B, Griffin JD, Tallman MS. Acute myeloid leukemia and acute promyelocytic leukemia. *Hematology Am Soc Hematol Educ Program* 2003:82–101.

21. Koreth J, Schlenk R, Kopecky KJ et al. Allogeneic stem cell transplantation for acute myeloid leukemia in first complete remission: systematic review and meta-analysis of prospective clinical trials. *JAMA* 2009;301:2349–61.

22. Slovak ML, Kopecky KJ, Cassileth PA et al. Karyotypic analysis predicts outcome of preremission and postremission therapy in adult acute myeloid leukemia: a Southwest Oncology Group/Eastern Cooperative Oncology Group Study. *Blood* 2000;96:4075–4083.

23. Burnett AK, Goldstone AH, Stevens RM et al. Randomised comparison of addition of autologous bone-marrow transplantation to intensive chemotherapy for acute myeloid leukaemia in first remission: results of MRC AML 10 trial. UK Medical Research Council Adult and Children's Leukaemia Working Parties. *Lancet* 1998;351:700–8.

24. Zittoun R, Jehn U, Fiere D et al. Alternating vs repeated postremission treatment in adult acute myelogenous leukemia: a randomized phase III study (AML6) of the EORTC Leukemia Cooperative Group. *Blood* 1989;73:896–906.

25. Harousseau JL, Cahn JY, Pignon B et al. Comparison of autologous bone marrow transplantation and intensive chemotherapy as postremission therapy in adult acute myeloid leukemia. The Groupe Ouest Est Leucemies Aigues Myeloblastiques (GOELAM). *Blood* 1997;90:2978–86.

26. Devine SM, Owzar K, Blum W et al. Phase II study of allogeneic transplantation for older patients with acute myeloid leukemia in first complete remission using a reduced-intensity conditioning regimen: results from Cancer and Leukemia Group B 100103 (Alliance for Clinical Trials in Oncology)/Blood and Marrow Transplant Clinical Trial Network 0502. *J Clin Oncol* 2015;33:4167–75.

27. Araki D, Wood BL, Othus M et al. Allogeneic hematopoietic cell transplantation for acute myeloid leukemia: time to move toward a minimal residual disease-based definition of complete remission? *J Clin Oncol* 2016;34:329–36.

28. Hourigan CS, Goswami M, Battiwalla M et al. When the minimal becomes measurable. *J Clin Oncol* 2016;34:2557–8.

29. Bensinger WI. Role of autologous and allogeneic stem cell transplantation in myeloma. *Leukemia* 2009;23:442–8.

30. Giles FJ, Keating A, Goldstone AH et al. Acute myeloid leukemia. *Hematology Am Soc Hematol Educ Program* 2002:73–110.

31. Cornelissen JJ, van Putten WL, Verdonck LF, Theobald M et al. Results of a HOVON/SAKK donor versus no-donor analysis of myeloablative HLA-identical sibling stem cell transplantation in first remission acute myeloid leukemia in young and middle-aged adults: benefits for whom? *Blood* 2007;109:3658–66.

32. Schmid C, Schleuning M, Schwerdtfeger R et al. Long-term survival in refractory acute myeloid leukemia after sequential treatment with chemotherapy and reduced-intensity conditioning for allogeneic stem cell transplantation. *Blood* 2006;108:1092–9.

33. Bejanyan N, Weisdorf DJ, Logan BR et al. Survival of patients with acute myeloid leukemia relapsing after allogeneic hematopoietic cell transplantation: a center for international blood and marrow transplant research study. *Biol Blood Marrow Transplant* 2015;21:454–9.

34. Xu W, Yang H, Liu Y et al. Oncometabolite 2-hydroxyglutarate is a competitive inhibitor of alpha-ketoglutarate-dependent dioxygenases. *Cancer Cell* 19:17–30.

35. Lu C, Ward PS, Kapoor GS et al. IDH mutation impairs histone demethylation and results in a block to cell differentiation. *Nature* 2012;483:474–8.

36. Figueroa ME, Abdel-Wahab O, Lu C et al. Leukemic IDH1 and IDH2 mutations result in a hypermethylation phenotype, disrupt TET2 function, and impair hematopoietic differentiation. *Cancer Cell* 2010;18:553–67.

37. Yen K, Travins J, Wang F et al. AG-221, a First-in-Class Therapy Targeting Acute Myeloid Leukemia Harboring Oncogenic IDH2 Mutations. *Cancer Discov* 2017;7: 478–93.

38. Stein EM, DiNardo CD, Pollyea DA et al. Enasidenib in mutant IDH2 relapsed or refractory acute myeloid leukemia. *Blood* 2017;130:722–31.

39. Shih A, Shank K, Meydan C et al. AG-221, a small molecule mutant IDH2 inhibitor, remodels the epigenetic state of IDH2-mutant cells and induces alterations in self-renewal/differentiation in IDH2-mutant AML model in vivo [abstract]. *Blood* 2014;124.

40. Fan B, Chen Y, Wang F et al. Pharmacokinetic/pharmacodynamic (PK/PD) evaluation of AG-221, a potent mutant IDH2 inhibitor, from a phase 1 trial of patients with IDH2 mutation-positive hematologic malignancies [abstract]. *Haematologica* 2015;100.

41. Marcucci G, Maharry K, Wu YZ et al. IDH1 and IDH2 gene mutations identify novel molecular subsets within de novo cytogenetically normal acute myeloid leukemia: a Cancer and Leukemia Group B study. *J Clin Oncol* 28:2348–55.

42. FDA. (2017) FDA granted regular approval to enasidenib for the treatment of relapsed or refractory AML. https://www.fda.gov/drugs/informationondrugs/approveddrugs/ucm569482.htm.

43. de Botton S, Pollyea D, Stein E et al. (2015) Clinical safety and activity of AG-120, a first-in-class, potent inhibitor of the IDH1 mutant protein, in a phase 1 study of patients with advanced idh1-mutant hematologic malignancies (poster presented at ASH20). https://learningcenter.ehaweb.org/eha/2015/20th/100704/stphane.debotton.clinical.safety.and.activity.of.ag-120.a.first-in-class.html.

44. Pfizer. (2017) Mylotarg (gemtuzumab ozogamicin) prescribing information.

45. Lo-Coco F et al. Retinoic acid and arsenic trioxide for acute promyelocytic leukemia. *N Engl J Med* 2013;369:111–121.

46. Ades, LA, et al. Very long-term outcome of acute promyelocytic leukemia after treatment with all-trans-retinoic acid and chemotherapy: the European APL Group experience. *Blood* 2010;115: 1690–1696.

47. Fenaux P, Chastang C, Chevret S et al. A randomized comparison of all transretinoic acid (ATRA) followed by chemotherapy and ATRA plus chemotherapy and the role of maintenance therapy in newly diagnosed acute promyelocytic leukemia. The European APL Group. *Blood* 1999;94:1192–1200.

48. Sanz MA, Martin G, Gonzalez M et al. Risk-adapted treatment of acute promyelocytic leukemia with all-trans-retinoic acid and anthracycline monochemotherapy: a multicenter study by the PETHEMA group. *Blood* 2004;103:1237–1243.

49. Powell BL, Moser B, Stock W et al. Arsenic trioxide improves event-free and overall survival for adults with acute promyelocytic leukemia: North American Leukemia Intergroup Study C9710. *Blood* 2010;116:3751–3757.

50. Ravandi F, Estey E, Jones D et al. Effective treatment of acute promyelocytic leukemia with all-trans-retinoic acid, arsenic trioxide, and gemtuzumab ozogamicin. *J Clin Oncol* 2009;27:504–510.

51. Gore SD, Gojo I, Sekeres MA et al. Single cycle of arsenic trioxide-based consolidation chemotherapy spares anthracycline exposure in the primary management of acute promyelocytic leukemia. *J Clin Oncol* 2010;28:1047–1053.

52. Mathews V, George B, Lakshmi KM et al. Single-agent arsenic trioxide in the treatment of newly diagnosed acute promyelocytic leukemia: durable remissions with minimal toxicity. *Blood* 2006;107:2627–2632.

53. Soignet SL, Frankel SR, Douer D et al. United States multicenter study of arsenic trioxide in relapsed acute promyelocytic leukemia. *J Clin Oncol* 2001;19:3852–3860.

**Treatment guidelines**

Döhner H, Estey E, Grimwade D et al. Diagnosis and management of AML in adults: 2017 ELN recommendations from an expert panel. *Blood* 2017;129:424–447.

O'Donnell MR, Tallman MS, Abboud CN et al. Acute myeloid leukemia, version 3.2107, NCCN Cllinical Practice Guidelines in Oncology. *J Natl Compr Canc Network* 2017; 15:926–957.

# 4 Supportive care

Treatment of acute myeloid leukemia (AML) involves repeated cycles of myelotoxic chemotherapy, resulting in prolonged cytopenia that requires intensive supportive care. Despite significant advances in supportive care over the last few decades, the treatment of AML is still associated with considerable morbidity and mortality, mostly related to infection.[1]

In the case of infection-related mortality, the emergence of multidrug resistant (MDR) organisms is a growing concern, particularly in developing economies[2], although increasingly this is now being recognized as a global phenomenon.[3] The presence of MDR bacteria adds significantly to morbidity and mortality in AML, and also contributes significantly to the cost of supportive care. In addition, proven (and suspected) invasive fungal infections occur in 14–28% of patients following induction chemotherapy[2,4,5] and are associated with early mortality.[6]

Strategies to improve outcomes, especially during induction therapy, include the following:

- mandatory hospitalization during chemotherapy
- use of granulocyte colony-stimulating factor (G-CSF) after chemotherapy
- prophylactic antibiotics
- prophylactic antifungals
- other supportive measures.

**Mandatory hospitalization.** During initial induction therapy, it is common practice to admit patients, typically for 3–4 weeks, until neutrophil levels recover, although data to support this approach are limited. In a pediatric population, a retrospective study by the Children's Oncology Group found no evidence that mandatory hospitalization reduced either systemic infections or treatment-related mortality.[1] Similar studies in adults have not been reported, but until more data become available, it seems reasonable to admit patients for at least the first 3–4 weeks of induction chemotherapy, unless easily accessible 24-hour supportive care is available. Limited data suggest that using a high-efficiency particulate-air-filtered facility is beneficial, and although this cannot be considered a standard recommendation, some indirect evidence suggests that this could reduce the rate of fungal infection.[7]

**Use of granulocyte colony-stimulating factor after chemotherapy.** Numerous studies, including meta-analyses, have consistently shown that the administration of G-CSF after completion of chemotherapy reduces the duration of neutropenia (typically 2–3 weeks) by 2–5 days. These studies have also shown that use of G-CSF reduces the duration of hospitalization, duration of fever and antibiotic use, and does not retard platelet recovery.[1,7] However, none of these beneficial effects has translated into improvements in overall survival. Based on current data, G-CSF is not recommended for all patients; however, its use can be considered in order to accelerate neutrophil recovery in patients with active or persistent infection, and those who are hemodynamically unstable secondary to infection.

**Prophylactic antibiotics.** Prophylactic use of quinolone antibiotics has been shown to reduce infection and mortality rates after chemotherapy.[8,9] Based on the available evidence, antibiotic prophylaxis after chemotherapy can be considered as standard care, and is a component of most international recommendations.[10] While quinolones are recommended on the basis of the available data, it is reasonable to review the treatment center's antibiogram to inform the choice of antibiotic.

**Prophylactic antifungal therapy.** The overall consensus, based on the available data, is that antifungal prophylaxis with posaconazole following chemotherapy is beneficial,[10] Micafungin is an alternative if azoles are contraindicated. Fungal prophylaxis typically consists of an anti-mold agent (e.g. posaconazole, micafungin or amphotericin) and should not be limited to anticandida cover, as would be achieved with fluconazole.

## Other supportive measures

**Hyperleukocytosis.** Leukapheresis, hydroxyurea and low-dose cytosine have all been suggested as treatment for hyperleukocytosis (white blood cell [WBC] count ≥ 100 000/mm$^3$ at presentation), although recent data suggest that none of these interventions reduce early treatment-related mortality in high-risk patients.[11] Patients with leukostasis (emergent organ dysfunction due to leukemic obstruction of vascular flow, especially in the lungs or brain) may benefit from emergency leukapheresis, although no controlled data are available to guide this decision. For younger patients, the current recommendation is to start standard 3 + 7 induction chemotherapy (see page 34), as soon as possible after diagnosis. For older patients who do not have proliferative AML/leuckocytosis, there does not appear to be any adverse effect from waiting until cytogenetic/genetic prognostication information is available in order to help guide the selection of therapy.

**Tumor lysis syndrome (TLS).** In comparison with acute lymphoblastic leukemia, the risk of TLS, and resultant hyperuricemia and renal failure, is relatively low in AML.[12] Among patients with AML, a WBC count at presentation of ≥100 000/mm$^3$ is considered high risk for developing TLS and hyperurcemia, and rasburicase should be considered for prophylaxis. For all other AML, hydration at 3 L/m$^2$, along with the administration of a xanthine oxidase inhibitor, such as allopurinol or febuxostat, over a short period of < 2 weeks (or based on response to therapy) is sufficient.[12]

**Venous catheter placement.** Although not part of any standard recommendation, good central venous access is considered essential for the administration of intensive chemotherapy and for allogeneic hematopoietic cell transplantation (alloHCT). The Hickman catheter is commonly preferred for alloSCT, while a peripherally inserted central venous catheter can also be considered for intensive chemotherapy. Although there are data suggesting that even with chemotherapy, the Hickman catheter is superior; this cannot be considered a standard recommendation based on these limited data.[13]

**Platelet infusion.** The agreed threshold for prophylactic platelet transfusion based on multiple studies is ≤ 10 000/mm$^3$.[7] However, a higher threshold should be considered in the presence of high-grade fever, mucositis and active bleeding. Recent data suggest that it is not acceptable to withhold prophylactic platelet infusion at this threshold when there is increased risk of bleeding, especially in the central nervous system.[14,15]

**Hemoglobin.** Hemoglobin levels should be maintained above 80 g/L following chemotherapy, although lower thresholds for red blood cell transfusions may reduce transfusion exposure without deleterious effects. Blood products should ideally be leukodepleted at source, in order to reduce the risk of febrile transfusion reaction and allo-immunization.

**Granulocyte infusion.** There is no evidence to support routine use of granulocyte infusion to reduce treatment-related infection and mortality.

**General hygiene.** Good personal hygiene is important, and particular attention should be paid to dental and perianal care during the post-chemotherapy neutropenic state.

While patients are often advised not to eat uncooked food such as salads and fruits (neutropenic diet), there is no evidence to support this.[16]

## Key points – supportive care

- The standard treatment of acute myeloid leukemia (AML) involves repeated cycles of myelotoxic chemotherapy, resulting in prolonged cytopenia that requires intensive supportive care.
- Treatment of AML is still associated with considerable morbidity and mortality, mostly related to infection; this risk is compounded by the emergence of bacteria with multidrug resistance.
- Standard practice is for patients to be hospitalized for induction chemotherapy until neutrophil recovery is achieved (3–4 weeks).
- Following chemotherapy, prophylactic antibiotics to prevent infection and reduce mortality rates is a standard recommendation; the choice of antibiotic should be informed by the local antibiogram. Prophylaxis with antifungals with both anti-mold and anticandida activity is beneficial.
- Attention to good hygiene, particularly dental and perianal care, is important.

## References


1. Sung L, Aplenc R, Alonzo TA et al. Effectiveness of supportive care measures to reduce infections in pediatric AML: a report from the Children's Oncology Group. *Blood* 2013;121:3573–7.

2. Philip C, George B, Ganapule A et al. Acute myeloid leukaemia: challenges and real world data from India. *Br J Haematol* 2015;170: 110–17.

3. Johnson AP, Woodford N. Global spread of antibiotic resistance: the example of New Delhi metallo-beta-lactamase (NDM)-mediated carbapenem resistance. *J Med Microbiol* 2013;62:499–513.

4. Barreto JN, Beach CL, Wolf RC et al. The incidence of invasive fungal infections in neutropenic patients with acute leukemia and myelodysplastic syndromes receiving primary antifungal prophylaxis with voriconazole. *Am J Hematol* 2013;88:283–8.

5. Gomes MZ, Mulanovich VE, Jiang Y et al. Incidence density of invasive fungal infections during primary antifungal prophylaxis in newly diagnosed acute myeloid leukemia patients in a tertiary cancer center, 2009 to 2011. *Antimicrob Agents Chemother* 2013;58:865–73.

6. Girmenia C, Micozzi A, Piciocchi A et al. Invasive fungal diseases during first induction chemotherapy affect complete remission achievement and long-term survival of patients with acute myeloid leukemia. *Leukemia Res* 2014;38:469–74.

7. Dohner H, Estey EH, Amadori S et al. Diagnosis and management of acute myeloid leukemia in adults: recommendations from an international expert panel, on behalf of the European LeukemiaNet. *Blood* 2010;115:453–74.

8. Leibovici L, Paul M, Cullen M et al. Antibiotic prophylaxis in neutropenic patients: new evidence, practical decisions. *Cancer* 2006;107:1743–51.

9. Gafter-Gvili A, Fraser A, Paul M, Leibovici L. Meta-analysis: antibiotic prophylaxis reduces mortality in neutropenic patients. *Ann Int Med* 2005;142:979–95.

10. Dohner H, Estey E, Grimwade D et al. Diagnosis and management of AML in adults: 2017 ELN recommendations from an international expert panel. *Blood* 2017;129:424–47.

11. Oberoi S, Lehrnbecher T, Phillips B et al. Leukapheresis and low-dose chemotherapy do not reduce early mortality in acute myeloid leukemia hyperleukocytosis: a systematic review and meta-analysis. *Leukemia Res* 2014;38:460–8.

12. Cairo MS, Coiffier B, Reiter A et al. Recommendations for the evaluation of risk and prophylaxis of tumour lysis syndrome (TLS) in adults and children with malignant diseases: an expert TLS panel consensus. *Br J Haematol* 2010;149:578–86.

13. Skaff ER, Doucette S, McDiarmid S et al. Vascular access devices in leukemia: a retrospective review amongst patients treated at the Ottawa Hospital with induction chemotherapy for acute leukemia. *Leuk Lymphoma* 2012;53:1090–5.

14. Wandt H, Schaefer-Eckart K, Wendelin K et al. Therapeutic platelet transfusion versus routine prophylactic transfusion in patients with haematological malignancies: an open-label, multicentre, randomised study. *Lancet* 2012;380:1309–16.

15. Stanworth SJ, Estcourt LJ, Powter G et al. A no-prophylaxis platelet-transfusion strategy for hematologic cancers. *N Engl J Med* 2013;368:1771–80.

16. Gardner A, Mattiuzzi G, Faderl S et al. Randomized comparison of cooked and noncooked diets in patients undergoing remission induction therapy for acute myeloid leukemia. *J Clin Oncol* 2008;26: 5684–8.

# 5 Prognosis and monitoring

Acute myeloid leukemia (AML) is a heterogeneous disorder; the current World Health Organization (WHO) classification (see Table 2.3) classifies the patient's 'risk' according to the molecular pathology (where this is known), which in turn informs the prognosis. Accurate prognostication is important when considering the risk versus benefit associated with different approaches to treatment (chemotherapy, novel targeted therapies, allogeneic hematopoietic cell transplant [alloHCT]), which are associated with different levels of early treatment-related mortality and risk of relapse. Prognostication requires evaluation of the following:[1]

- pre-treatment risk based on:
  - age
  - comorbidities
  - cytogenetic and molecular analysis
- post-treatment parameters: measurable residual disease (MRD) monitoring.

## Age

Multiple studies have established age as an important and independent adverse risk factor; in particular, older patients (> 60 years) have dismal outcomes with conventional treatment. Table 5.1 summarizes data from a retrospective analysis of the combined adverse effects of older age and poor performance status on mortality risk. This and other studies have also identified a positive correlation between increasing age and adverse cytogenetic and molecular markers, and with increased incidence of multidrug resistance to chemotherapy.[2, 3] Performance status and comorbidities should also be considered alongside age when deciding on the intensity of treatment to offer older patients with AML.

TABLE 5.1

**Influence of age and performance status on mortality risk with early induction chemotherapy**

| ECOG PS | Age (years) | | | |
|---|---|---|---|---|
| | < 56 | 56–65 | 66–75 | > 75 |
| 0 | 2* | 11 | 12 | 14 |
| 1 | 3 | 5 | 16 | 18 |
| 2 | 2 | 18 | 31 | 50 |
| 3 | 0 | 29 | 47 | 82 |

*Values are percentage risk.
ECOG PS, Eastern Cooperative Oncology Group performance status
Modified from Appelabaum et al., 2006.[3]

## Comorbidities

Comorbidities affect the morbidity and mortality risks of treatments and therefore inform treatment choices. For example, conventional anthracycline-based induction chemotherapy would not be suitable for a patient with a history of ischemic or congestive heart disease. Patients may also develop consequences of AML that influence the treatment strategy, such as severe sepsis.

## Cytogenetic and molecular signatures

Cytogenetics and the molecular signature have become the cornerstone of risk stratification in AML.[1,4] The risk groups based on karyotyping used by the cooperative groups (Cancer and Leukemia Group B, SWOG and the Eastern Cooperative Oncology Group) are illustrated in Table 5.2.[5] Prognostic assignment differs slightly among North American and European groups but the basic premise is shared. Additional parameters such as age, white blood cell count at diagnosis, presence of certain gene mutations and response to induction chemotherapy can influence prognosis, while the type of consolidation therapy could potentially alter the predicted outcomes, as discussed in Chapter 4.

The last decade has seen an explosion in our understanding of the molecular genetics of AML, and the recognition that several of these

TABLE 5.2

**Risk group stratification based on cytogenetics at diagnosis**

| Risk category | Favorable | Intermediate | Adverse |
|---|---|---|---|
| Proportion of patients | 10–15 | 65–75 | 15–20 |
| Cytogenetic features | t(15;17)<br>t(8;21)<br>inv(16)<br>t(16;16) | Normal karyotype<br>del(9q)<br>–y<br>del(12p)<br>Trisomy 8<br>t(9;11) | Abnormal 5 or 7<br>inv(3q)<br>del(20q)<br>del(21q)<br>t(9;22)<br>t(6;9)<br>Non-t(9;11) 11q23 abnormalities with MLL rearrangements<br>Complex cytogenetics (≥ 3 clonal abnormalities) |
| Probability of relapse (%)[a] | 25 | 50 | > 70 |
| 4-year survival probability (%)[a] | 70 | 40–50 | < 20 |

del, deletion; inv, inversion; t, tranlocation.
Modified from Cassileth et al., 1998[5] and Lowenberg et al., 2003.[6]

abnormalities (not previously recognized on a conventional karyotype), either alone or in combination, have a significant bearing on prognosis. The numerous genetic abnormalities seen in AML are summarized in the recent European LeukemiaNet (ELN) guidelines.[1] The ELN has recently revised the risk stratification groups for AML on the basis of the genetic abnormalities detected by conventional karyotyping and molecular techniques (see Table 2.4). Many of these mutations are context specific in both their occurrence and impact on clinical outcomes. For example:

- *ASXL-1* mutations occur more commonly in older patients and are also associated with poor prognosis
- *NPM1* mutation is associated with a good prognosis only in the absence of other high-risk mutations such as *FLT3* internal tandem duplication (*FLT3*-ITD) with high allelic ratio.

Molecular markers can be used within the cytogenetically defined risk groups to further refine the prognostic risk, and may even be useful in deciding the optimal consolidation therapy, as illustrated in the following two scenarios.

- In the large cohort of patient with cytogenetically normal karyotype, mutation analysis in *NPM1* and *FLT3* can help distinguish three subsets:
  - *NPM1*+ / *FLT3*-ITD– (without adverse-risk genetic lesions) is associated with good prognosis; consolidation with chemotherapy alone may be considered, as for a cytogenetic favorable-risk group (note that the ELN 2017 update includes *FLT3*-ITD with a 'low' mutated to wild-type ratio [< 0.5] in this group)
  - *NPM1*+ / *FLT3*-ITD+ is associated with intermediate risk
  - *NPM1*– / *FLT3*-ITD+ may be considered as high risk; allogeneic HCT may therefore be offered at first complete remission (CR1).

  The impact of these combinations on event-free and overall survival has been shown by a retrospective analysis of two consecutive AML Study Group trials, as illustrated in Figure 5.1.[7]
- Within the cytogenetically favorable-risk group, the presence of a *KIT* mutation is associated with poor prognosis and may therefore identify a subset of favorable-risk patients for whom allogeneic HCT can be considered in CR1.[8]

With the increasing use of high-throughput molecular analysis, clinicians can look forward to the identification of well-defined biologic entities to enhance prognostication in AML. The identification of novel markers beyond prognostication may also help identify subsets of patients who may benefit from therapies with specific molecular targets. This is best illustrated by the recent success demonstrated with the *FLT3* inhibitor midostaurin, described on

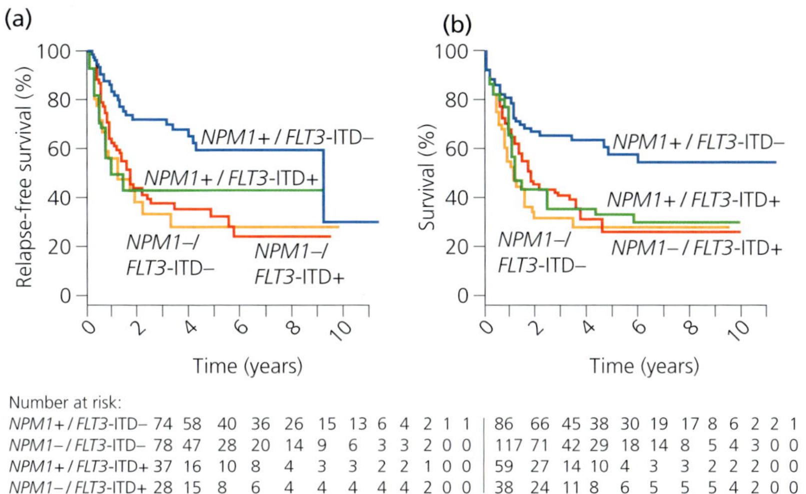


Number at risk:

| | (a) | | | | | | | | | | | | (b) | | | | | | | | | | | |
|---|---|---|---|---|---|---|---|---|---|---|---|---|---|---|---|---|---|---|---|---|---|---|---|---|
| *NPM1+ / FLT3*-ITD– | 74 | 58 | 40 | 36 | 26 | 15 | 13 | 6 | 4 | 2 | 1 | 1 | 86 | 66 | 45 | 38 | 30 | 19 | 17 | 8 | 6 | 2 | 2 | 1 |
| *NPM1– / FLT3*-ITD– | 78 | 47 | 28 | 20 | 14 | 9 | 6 | 3 | 3 | 2 | 0 | 0 | 117 | 71 | 42 | 29 | 18 | 14 | 8 | 5 | 4 | 3 | 0 | 0 |
| *NPM1+ / FLT3*-ITD+ | 37 | 16 | 10 | 8 | 4 | 3 | 3 | 2 | 2 | 1 | 0 | 0 | 59 | 27 | 14 | 10 | 4 | 3 | 3 | 2 | 2 | 2 | 0 | 0 |
| *NPM1– / FLT3*-ITD+ | 28 | 15 | 8 | 6 | 4 | 4 | 4 | 4 | 4 | 2 | 0 | 0 | 38 | 24 | 11 | 8 | 6 | 5 | 5 | 5 | 4 | 2 | 0 | 0 |

**Figure 5.1** Impact of *NPM1* and *FLT3*-ITD mutations on (a) relapse-free survival and (b) overall survival ($p = 0.01$ for both). ITD, internal tandem duplications. Adapted from Dohner et al., 2005.[7]

page 36.[9] Similar targeted therapies are being evaluated for *IDH1*, *IDH2* and *KMT2A* mutations, as discussed in Chapter 6.[1]

## Measurable residual disease monitoring

Patients who do not achieve CR after the first cycle of induction chemotherapy are considered to be at high risk for relapse. The presence of MRD after completion of induction and consolidation chemotherapy despite morphological remission has significant prognostic implication. MRD can be measured using multiparameter flow cytometry (MFC; successful in > 90% of cases) or real-time quantitative polymerase chain reaction (RT-qPCR) assays where a molecular lesion has been identified. MFC requires substantial technical expertise, and interpretation is partially subjective so it has been difficult to establish inter-laboratory standardization. RT-qPCR can only be used if a molecular marker has been identified (< 60% of cases) and also has challenges in standardization; more importantly, the oligoclonal nature of AML at diagnosis (see pages 14–15) means that a negative reading must be interpreted with caution. Despite these challenges, several studies have established the role of MRD in the accurate prognosis of outcomes when performed after induction and consolidation therapy and before alloHCT.[1] MRD monitoring is uniquely beneficial for high-risk APL patients in CR1.

Detection of rising MRD has been shown to accurately predict relapse.[10] Studies are currently investigating whether intervention based on such information can improve clinical outcomes in AML.[1]

Next-generation sequencing (NGS) provides a new means for MRD monitoring that can potentially be applied to all cases of AML and may help to accurately identify molecular subclones, with the potential to improve prognostication and treatment by offering novel targeted therapies directed at smaller subclones that may not have been detected by other conventional molecular techniques.[10] Currently, NGS is investigational for diagnosis, MRD detection and sequential MRD monitoring and is not yet a component of standard of care.

**Key points – prognosis and monitoring**

- Accurate prognostication is important when considering the risk versus benefit associated with different approaches to treatment.
- The World Health Organization system classifies patients' 'risk' based on molecular pathology.
- Age is an important and independent adverse risk factor, and older patients (> 60 years) have particularly dismal outcomes with conventional treatment. Age and certain cytogenetic or molecular abnormalities increase the risk of multidrug resistance to chemotherapy.
- Understanding of the molecular genetics of acute myeloid leukemia has increased in the last decade, and several mutations, either alone or in combination, have been shown to have a significant bearing on prognosis. European LeukemiaNet includes these genetic abnormalities in its risk stratification.
- Molecular markers can be used within the cytogenetically defined risk groups to further refine the prognostic risk and may influence the choice of consolidation therapy.
- The presence of measurable residual disease after induction chemotherapy indicates a high risk of relapse.

## References

1. Dohner H, Estey E, Grimwade D et al. Diagnosis and management of AML in adults: 2017 ELN recommendations from an international expert panel. *Blood* 2017;129:424–47.

2. Appelbaum FR, Rowe JM, Radich J, Dick JE. Acute myeloid leukemia. *Hematology Am Soc Hematol Educ Program* 2001:62–86.

3. Appelbaum FR, Gundacker H, Head DR et al. Age and acute myeloid leukemia. *Blood* 2006;107:3481–5.

4. Slovak ML, Kopecky KJ, Cassileth PA et al. Karyotypic analysis predicts outcome of preremission and postremission therapy in adult acute myeloid leukemia: a Southwest Oncology Group/Eastern Cooperative Oncology Group Study. *Blood* 2000;96:4075–83.

5. Cassileth PA, Harrington DP, Appelbaum FR et al. Chemotherapy compared with autologous or allogeneic bone marrow transplantation in the management of acute myeloid leukemia in first remission. *N Engl J Med* 1998;339:1649–56.

6. Lowenberg B, Griffin JD, Tallman MS. Acute myeloid leukemia and acute promyelocytic leukemia. *Hematology Am Soc Hematol Educ Program* 2003:82–101.

7. Dohner K, Schlenk RF, Habdank M et al. Mutant nucleophosmin (NPM1) predicts favorable prognosis in younger adults with acute myeloid leukemia and normal cytogenetics: interaction with other gene mutations. *Blood* 2005;106:3740–6.

8. Paschka P, Marcucci G, Ruppert AS et al. Adverse prognostic significance of KIT mutations in adult acute myeloid leukemia with inv(16) and t(8;21): a Cancer and Leukemia Group B Study. *J Clin Oncol* 2006;24:3904–11.

9. Stone RM, Mandrekar SJ, Sanford BL et al. Midostaurin plus chemotherapy for acute myeloid leukemia with a FLT3 mutation. *N Engl J Med* 2017;377:454–64.

10. Grimwade D, Freeman SD. Defining minimal residual disease in acute myeloid leukemia: which platforms are ready for 'prime time'? *Blood* 2014;124:3345–55.

# 6 Research directions

The expanded genetic characterization of acute myeloid leukemia (AML) at diagnosis is a critical advance in the last 5 years and is influencing both treatment and patient selection for standard therapy and clinical trials in AML. While the karyotype remains key in prognostication, molecular profiling represents a paradigm shift for both research and the clinical management of AML. Molecular testing is destined to become an essential part of the initial characterization of patients with AML.

## Drugs in late-stage development

As described in Chapter 3, four new treatments for AML were recently approved, three of which are molecularly targeted products, marking a turning point in the treatment of AML. Several targeted agents are currently in the late stages of clinical development, as described below, and many more approaches are being explored (see Table 6.1). Many of these products in development have been awarded breakthrough status by the US Food and Drug Administration (FDA), recognizing the lack of effective treatments for patients who are not eligible for intensive chemotherapy and hematopoietic cell transplantation (HCT), and those with relapsed or refractory disease, for whom the prognosis is poor.

**FLT3 inhibitors.** In addition to midostaurin, several other FLT3 inhibitors are currently in trials.[1]

***Crenolanib*** inhibits *FLT3* internal tandem repeat (*FLT3*-ITD) and *FLT3* tyrosine kinase domain (*FLT3*-TKD) mutations in the active conformation but has little activity against cKIT; this is expected to avoid the myelosuppression seen with other FLT3 inhibitors that have been shown to inhibit KIT. The addition of crenolanib to standard 3 + 7 induction therapy in patients with newly diagnosed AML resulted in 88% complete response rate (CR), with no unexpected toxicities.[2]

TABLE 6.1

**Novel therapies in clinical development for the treatment of acute myeloid leukemia (AML)**

**Protein kinase inhibitors**

- FLT3 inhibitors (quizartinib, gilteritnib, crenolanib, sorafenib)
- KIT inhibitors
- PI3K/AKT/mTOR inhibitors
- Aurora and polo-like kinase inhibitors, CDK4/6 inhibitors, CHK1, WEE1 and MPS1 inhibitors
- SRC and HCK inhibitors
- Syk inhibitors (entospletinib)

**Epigenetic modulators**

- New DNA methyltransferase inhibitors (SGI-110, oral azacitidine)
- Histone deacetylase (HDAC) inhibitors (pracinostat)
- IDH1 and IDH2 inhibitors
- DOT1L inhibitors
- BET-bromodomain inhibitors

**Mitochondrial inhibitors**

- Bcl-2 (venetoclax), Bcl-xL and Mcl-1 inhibitors

**Therapies targeting oncogenic proteins**

- NPM1 targeting
- Hedgehog inhibitors

**Antibodies and immunotherapies**

- Monoclonal antibodies against CD33, CD44, CD47, CD123, CLEC12A
- Antibody–drug conjugates (e.g. SGN33A/vadastuximab talirine*)
- Bispecific T-cell engagers (BiTEs) and dual-affinity re-targeting molecules (DARTs)

**Antibodies and immunotherapies**

- Chimeric antigen-receptor (CAR) T-cells or genetically engineered T-cell receptor (TCR) T-cells targeting CD123 (e.g. UCART123*), CD33, LeY, CLL-1

(CONTINUED)

TABLE 6.1 (CONTINUED)

**Novel therapies in clinical development for the treatment of acute myeloid leukemia**

**Antibodies and immunotherapies**

- Immune checkpoint inhibitors (PD-1/PD-L1, CTLA-4)
- Anti-KIR antibody (endpoint not reached in Phase II study of irilumab for maintenance treatment)
- Vaccines (e.g. WT1)
- Novel approached to allogeneic stem cell or effector cell transplantation approaches

**Therapies targeting AML environment**

- CXCR4 and CXCL12 antagonists
- Anti-angiogenic therapies

Adapted from Döhner H et al. Diagnosis and management of acute myeloid leukemia in adults: 2017 recommendations from an international expert panel, on behalf of the European LeukemiaNet. *Blood*. Epub 2016 Nov 28.

*Product currently on FDA clinical hold because of safety concerns.

***Quizartinib (AC220).*** A non-randomized Phase II study reported a remission rate of 44% and median overall survival (OS) of 23 weeks in patients with *FLT3*-ITD-mutated AML that had relapsed or was refractory to second-line treatment or relapsed following HCT in a non-randomized Phase II study.[3] Quizartinib is being investigated across multiple lines of treatment, including induction and consolidation chemotherapy, as a maintenance therapy for patients in first remission after chemotherapy, and for salvage therapy.[4]

***Gilteritinib*** is also being evaluated across multiple lines of treatment in patients with FLT3-positive AML, including for maintenance treatment following chemotherapy or HCT, first-line treatment, and in comparison with salvage chemotherapy in patients with relapsed disease. Gilteritinib is thought to be more potent than midostaurin, as it also targets the kinase AXL, which is thought to contribute to the resistance seen with other FLT3 inhibitors.[5]

***Sorafenib*** (which is already used to treat renal cell carcinoma and hepatocellular carcinoma) has shown promising results in various lines of treatment.[6] A Phase II single-arm study in which sorafenib was added to standard induction/consolidation and continued as maintenance in elderly patients (> 60 years) with *FLT3*-ITD or *FLT3*-TKD mutations reported CR or CR with incomplete blood count recovery (CRi) in 69% of patients and 1-year OS of 62% (*FLT3*-ITD) and 71% (*FLT3*-TKD) at a median follow-up of 28.3 months. Median OS was 12.5 and 9.0 months, respectively, and disease-free survival was 15.0 and 16.2 months, respectively. Sorafenib has also been explored as monotherapy and in combination with chemotherapy in patients with relapsed *FLT3*-mutated AML, before or after transplant, with profound and sustained remissions being observed in some patients.

**Hypomethylating agents** in development include guadecitabine and oral azacitidine. Decitabine and subcutaneous azacitidine are already used for the treatment of myelodysplastic syndrome and AML. Guadecitabine is a dinucleotide of decitabine and deoxyguanosine, which protects decitabine from degradation in the intracellular compartment. Phase II studies have reported increases in response rates compared with historical data, and promising median OS in responders. Oral azacitidine is currently being evaluated as maintenance therapy for patients with AML who are not eligible for HCT, and as maintenance therapy in the post-transplant setting for patients with advanced myeloid malignancies.

**Histone deacetylase inhibitors.** Pracinostat is an oral histone deacetylase inhibitor that is being evaluated in combination with azacitidine for the treatment of newly diagnosed AML in older patients (≥ 75 years) who are unfit for intensive chemotherapy (because of age or comorbidities).[7] A Phase II study in this population showed a median OS of 19.1 months and a CR rate of 42% (21 of 50 patients), compared with OS of 10.4 months and CR of 19.5 with for azacitidine alone in a Phase III study.

**The bcl-2 inhibitor** venetoclax is already licensed for use in chronic lymphocytic leukemia and is now being evaluated in AML. Activity was limited as monotherapy in AML but much better response rates were seen in combination with hypomethylating agents (decitabine or azactidine) in older patients (≥ 65 years) who were not eligible for induction chemotherapy: 70–75% of patients achieved CR or CRi.[9] Venetoclax is also being evaluated in combination with low-dose cytarabine in a non-randomized open-label Phase I/II study in elderly patients (≥ 65 years) with treatment-naïve AML who not eligible for intensive chemotherapy.

**E-selectin inhibitors.** GMI-1271 is a novel antagonist of E-selectin, an adhesion molecule expressed in AML cells that has been shown to enhance responses to chemotherapy. A Phase II study of GMI-1271 in combination with cytarabine plus mitoxantrone and etoposide in patients (aged >60 years) reported a CR/CRi rate of 75% in those with treatment-naïve AML and 67% in those with secondary AML.[10]

## Novel immunotherapies

The FDA has recently approved two novel immunologic therapies for malignancies of B-lymphocytes: chimeric antigen receptor (CAR) T-cell products that target CD19 (by Novartis for acute lymphoblastic leukemia; by KITE for non-Hodgkin lymphoma). In both cases, autologous B-cells are collected from the patient by apheresis, genetically engineered to target CD19, then infused back into the patient. High response rates and durable remissions have been reported in patients with highly refractory disease. Whether the method of CAR targeting can be successfully applied to other hematologic cancers such as AML remains to be seen. Clearly, there are unique features of the target in B-lymphocytes (CD19; in particular, its lack of expression in other tissues beyond B-cells). A number of other CAR immune cells targeting other molecules are in development, including in AML.

The challenges in drug development in this area are highlighted by recent reports from Cellectis on its 'off the shelf' CD123-CAR T-cell trial for AML and the related disorder of blastic plasmacytoid dendritic cell neoplasm (BPDCN). CD123 is highly expressed in BPDCN and in early myeloid cells. Treatment of two patients with the CD123-CAR T-cell product (UCART123) resulted in cytokine release syndrome and one death.

Nevertheless, studies of cellular therapies, including CAR-T and natural killer (NK) cells, and antibody products targeting CD123, CD33 and other markers, are of interest. New approaches to treatment include antibody–drug conjugates (ADC) and novel antibody-based approaches using bispecific T-cell engagers (BiTEs) and dual-affinity re-targeting (DART) molecules, which bind to CD3 on T-lymphocytes and CD33 on myeloid blasts, thereby directing activated immune cells to malignant cells. Studies with cellular therapies and other antibody-based therapies are of great interest and promise in AML, including with CAR-T or NK cells, and likewise with antibody products targeting CD123, CD33 or other markers of interest. Included among these are new ADCs and novel antibody-based approaches using BiTEs or DARTs designed to direct activated immune cells to malignant cells (i.e. dual affinity for CD3 on T-lymphocytes and CD33 on myeloid blasts).

## A new era for clinical trials in AML?

Recent experience with enasidenib, approved on the basis of data from patients specifically with *IDH2* mutations, challenges the dogma that large randomized controlled trials showing survival benefit in a general AML population are required for approval. The approval of enasidenib was based on data from a single-arm phase 1/2 monotherapy trial involving only 199 patients; historical data were used for the control. This approval reflects the regulatory agencies' recognition of the challenges of evaluating new treatments in relatively rare subtypes of a disease; similar approvals have been seen across a range of oncology (hematologic and solid tumors) in recent years. Trials of new targeted agents are also likely to be in small, clearly identified patient populations.

**Beat AML** is a new approach to clinical trials, begun in late 2016 and sponsored by the Leukemia & Lymphoma Society.[11] The aim is to quickly and comprehensively genetically characterize older patients (> 60 years) with previously untreated AML and to treat with novel targeted therapy on the basis of the genetic result. Within a week of diagnosis, patients will be assigned to one of nine groups with targetable molecular aberrations (Table 6.2). Each group is treated with unique therapy designed for that molecular aberration. Patients who have more favorable clinical outcomes with conventional

TABLE 6.2

**Potential targetable molecular/cytogenetic groups in Beat AML version 1.0[11]**

| |
|---|
| CBF alterations |
| *NPM1* mutation (no *FLT3* mutation) |
| *MLL* balanced rearrangement or *MLL-PTD* |
| *IDH2* mutations |
| *IDH1* mutations |
| *TP53* mutations |
| *FLT3* mutations |
| *TET2/WT1* mutations |
| *DNMT3A* mutations |

CBF, core binding factor; PTD, partial tandem duplication.

chemotherapy (such as those with core binding factor rearrangements or an *NPM1* mutation without an *FLT3* mutation) are assigned 3 + 7-based treatment in combination with an investigational agent. Patients with poor long-term outcomes and lower remission rates with conventional chemotherapy (such as those with a *p53* mutation) receive less intensive therapy. Two examples of treatments in these poor-risk subsets are hypomethylating agent in combination with novel therapy, and monotherapy with an investigational agent followed by lower-intensity treatment (if no response is observed during the monotherapy window). Hopefully, such an approach will quickly identify promising agents and speed up drug approvals in AML. Subsequent iterations of the trial (e.g. 'version 2.0' and beyond) will include agents for other targets and possibly combinations of novel drugs.

Of critical importance to the Beat AML trial, as well as for trials of treatments, is the need to achieve disease control in order to facilitate the opportunity for alloHCT for eligible patients. Even in the era of molecular targeted treatment, alloHCT remains the best tool available for the prevention of relapse.

**Key points – research directions**

- A wide range of targeted agencies for the treatment of acute myeloid leukemia (AML) are currently in the late stages of development, including FLT3 inhibitors (crenolanib, quizartinib, gilteritinib, sorafenib), hypomethylating agents (guadecitabine, oral azacitidine), the histone deacetylase inhibitor pracinostat, the blc-2 inhibitor venetoclax and the E-selectin inhibitor GM-1271.
- Immunologic therapies, antibody–drug conjugates and antibody-based approaches are also being explored in AML.
- The approval of enasidenib based on single-arm Phase I/II data is challenging the dogma that large randomized controlled trials in a general AML population are required. Trials of new targeted agents are likely to be in small, clearly defined patients with subtypes of AML.
- The Beat AML trial is using early and comprehensive genetic characterization to assign patients to one of nine groups with targetable molecular aberrations, each receiving a tailored treatment. This approach will hopefully speed up the development of promising agents.
- Key to all approaches to the treatment of AML is the need to achieve disease control, and continued consideration of allogeneic hematopoietic cell transplantation when feasible.

## References


1. Saygin C and Carraway HE. Emerging therapies for acute myeloid leukemia. *J Hematol Oncol* 2017;10:93 doi.org/10.1186/s13045-017-0463-6

2. Wang E, Stone R, Collins R et al. Variant FLT3 mutations can be eradicated by cytarabine/anthracycline/crenolanib induction in adult patients with newly diagnosed FLT3 (ITD/TKD) mutant AML. Presented at: 2017 EHA Congress; June 22-25, 2017; Madrid, Spain. Abstract P552.

3. Döhner H et al. Diagnosis and management of acute myeloid leukemia in adults: 2017 recommendations from an international expert panel, on behalf of the European LeukemiaNet. *Blood* 2017;129:424–447.

4. Hills RK, Gammon G, Trone D, Burnett AK. Quizartinib significantly improves overall survival in FLT3-ITD positive AML patients relapsed after stem cell transplantation or after failure of salvage chemotherapy: A comparison with historical AML database (UK NCRI data). *Blood* 2015;126:2557.

5. Daiichi-Sankyo 2016. http://www.daiichisankyo.com/media_investors/media_relations/press_releases/detail/006529.html Last accessed 5 December 2017.

6. http://www.pmlive.com/pharma_news/astellas_extends_phase_iii_programme_for_rydapt_rival_gilteritinib_1203055 Last accessed 5 December 2017.

7. Antar A, Otrock ZK, El-Cheikh J et al. Inhibition of FLT3 in AML: a focus on sorafenib. *Bone Marrow Transplant* 2017;52:344–351.

8. Helsinn 2016. https://www.helsinn.com/news-and-events/helsinn-group-and-mei-pharma-enter-strategic-agreement-for-the-development-of-pracinostat-for-the-treatment-myeloid-leukemia-and-other-diseases/ Last accessed 5 December 2017.

9. Courtney DiNardo C, Pollyea D, Pratz K et al. A phase 1b study of venetoclax (ABT-199/GDC-0199) in combination with decitabine or azacitidine in treatment-naive patients with acute myelogenous leukemia who are ≥ to 65 years and not eligible for standard induction therapy. *Blood* 2015;126:327.

10. DeAngelo DJ, Jonas BA, Liesveld J, et al. GMI-1271, a novel E-selectin antagonist, in combination with chemotherapy in relapsed/refractory AML. *J Clin Oncol* 2017;15(suppl): Abstract 2520.

11. Study Seeks New AML therapies. *Cancer Discov* 2016;6:1297–98.

# Useful resources

## UK

**Bloodwise**
39–40 Eagle Street, London, WC1R 4TH
Tel: +44(0)20 7504 2200
Support Line (UK): 0808 2080 888
www.bloodwise.org.uk

**Cancer Research UK**
PO BOX 1561
Oxford OX4 9GZ
Tel: +44 (0)300 123 1022
supporter.services@cancer.org.uk
www.cancerresearchuk.org

**Leuka**
52 Portland Place
London W1B 1NH
Tel: +44 (0)20 7299 0722
info@leuka.org.uk
www.leuka.org.uk

**Leukaemia Cancer Society**
118 Myddleton Rd
London N22 8NQ
Tel: +44 (0)20 8374 4821
info@leukaemiacancersociety.org
www.leukaemiacancersociety.org

**Leukaemia Care**
Tel (UK) : 01905 755977
Careline: 0808 8010 444
info@leukaemiacare.org.uk
www.leukaemiacare.org.uk

**Leukaemia & Myeloma Research UK**
Unit 127, North Mersey Business Centre
Woodward Road, Knowsley Industrial
Park, Liverpool L33 7UY
Tel (UK): 0800 368 7309
cs@leukaemiamyelomaresearchuk.org
www.leukaemiamyelomaresearchuk.org

## USA

**Leukemia Research Foundation**
91 Waukegan Road, Suite 105
Northfield, IL 60093-2744
Tel: + 847 424 0600
email via website
www.allbloodcancers.org

**The Leukemia & Lymphoma Society**
3 International Drive, Suite 200
Rye Brook, NY 10573
Tel: + 914 949 5213
www.lls.org/beat-aml

## International

**Leukaemia Foundation (Australia)**
Toll-free: 1 800 620 420
www.leukaemia.org.au
info@leukaemia.org.au

**Leukemia and Lymphoma Society of Canada**
2 Lansing Square, Suite 804
Toronto, ON M2J 4P8
Tel: +1 877 668 8326
www.llscanada.org

# Index

**Notes:**

**Notes:**

**Notes:**

**Notes:**

**Notes:**